YOGA
of the
heart

YOGA of the *heart*

Ten Ethical Principles for Gaining Limitless Growth, Confidence, and Achievement

Alice Christensen

AMERICAN
Y · O · G · A
ASSOCIATION

Produced by The Philip Lief Group, Inc.

Daybreak® Books
An Imprint of Rodale Books
New York, New York

Cover Designer: Lynn N. Gano
Cover Photographer: Evelyn England, SAGE, Sarasota, Florida
Interior Designer: Faith Hague
Interior Illustrators: Patricia Rockwood, Alice Christensen

Library of Congress Cataloging-in-Publication Data
Christensen, Alice.
 Yoga of the heart : ten ethical principles for gaining limitless
 growth, confidence, and achievement / Alice Christensen.
 p. cm.
 ISBN 0–87596–429–X hardcover
 1. Yoga, Hatha. 2. Self-care, Health—Popular works.
 I. Title.
 RA781.7.C53 1998
 613.7'046—dc21   97–49103

Distributed in the book trade by St. Martin's Press

2 4 6 8 10 9 7 5 3 1 hardcover

OUR PURPOSE

*"We publish books that empower
people's minds and spirits."*

To my two great teachers:
Rama of Haridwar and Kashmir, and
Lakshmanjoo of Kashmir

The heart has its reasons, which reason knows nothing of.

BLAISE PASCAL

CONTENTS

ACKNOWLEDGMENTS

I wish to thank the staff of the American Yoga Association for their support and assistance during the preparation of this book, particularly Pattie Cerar, Linda Gajevski, Stephen R. Grant, Cynthia Ingalls, Nancy Leland, and Patricia Rockwood.

FOREWORD

In the summer of 1988, when I arrived in Kashmir to visit my teacher, the great Lakshmanjoo—a trip I had been making every summer for nearly twenty years—he was in deep despair. Kashmir, the northernmost state in India, was in turmoil, torn by rival political factions and military insurgents. Although Lakshmanjoo's own life and property were not directly threatened by this conflict, an American couple who had lived and studied with him for many years were falsely accused of being smugglers and had been deported.

The loss of these and other precious relationships in his later years (Lakshmanjoo was then eighty-three years old), combined with the warlike atmosphere in his homeland, brought him very near to death. By the time I reached him that summer, he had shaved his head (the traditional sign of impending departure from this world), had begun to refuse food, and had stopped speaking. In his grief, he had lost all impetus to continue living.

I refused to believe that this great teacher's work in the world was over. Lakshmanjoo had lived his entire life in pursuit of Yogic realization and was known throughout India for his mastery of the philosophy of Kashmir Shaivism and for his respected translations of the works of Abhinavagupta, a great teacher of Shaivism in the tenth century. One of Lakshman-joo's most well-known acquaintances was the late Indira Gandhi, India's former prime minister, who often traveled to Kashmir to consult with him during her lifetime.

The philosophy of Kashmir Shaivism had intrigued me from the very beginning of my study of Yoga. Everything in the universe, according to this thought, has both male and female qualities. Although it is impossible to describe these qualities exactly, some words that could be associated with the male principle are consciousness, energy, mind, and potentiality. The female principle could be described in terms such as manifestation, movement, and form. Many other Yogic philosophies, such as Vedanta, recognize only the male principle, saying that the female aspect—that is, the manifest world—is unreal; that is why you often see pictures of ascetics attempting to negate their bodies through suffering and self-denial. They are attempting to prove to themselves that the world, or the female aspect, is not important.

Kashmir Shaivism, on the other hand, recognizes that these male and female principles are an equal partnership, that they are so interdependent, they cannot be separated. They are, in fact, one thing. The feeling of attraction between them creates the immense complexity of the universe that we enjoy and celebrate.

Also unlike other philosophies, Kashmir Shaivism is based on emotion rather than intellect. In fact, Shaivism says that intellectual understanding by itself will never lead us to "realization," the summit of Yoga, because it blocks our ability to experience the full power of that male/female consciousness in ourselves.

In this book, I present this concept of the male/female consciousness that resides in you by using a fantasy picture of a second body, the spiritual body. I pretend that its limbs are various emotions and feelings, and its voice is intuition. In order for you to hear this voice of intuition speak, the intellect and ego must fall silent.

In Yogic texts, this second spiritual body is often evoked with the image of a heart. Even in casual speech, we often say that we are speaking "from the heart" when talking about some deep emotional or spiritual experience. When your spiritual body reveals itself and joins with your physical consciousness, the result is a powerful, enlightened individual who has not one heart but two with which to celebrate spiritual awareness. Our hands are the active, creative expression of our hearts, and so I have used a photograph of hands on the cover of this book to symbolize the meeting of your two hearts. This joining of the spiritual and physical hearts is what is meant by the title of this book.

The easiest way to invite your spiritual body to reveal itself is through the practice of Yogic ethics. The word *ethics* often implies a moralistic or religious prescription. Kashmir Shaivism uses this term in a different way. Ethics are the attitudes and behaviors that help you to welcome the spiritual being. They smooth the path to realizing your full potential.

I have chosen ten ethics that represent a part of those discussed in classical Yogic texts. These are done even before the exercises, breathing techniques, and meditation that are more familiar to us in the West. The ten ethics of Yoga that I will introduce in this book are Nonviolence, Truthfulness, Nonstealing, Celibacy, Nonhoarding, Purity, Contentment, Tolerance, Study, and Remembrance. I will talk more about how to approach these ethics as a whole in chapter 3, and each ethic will be discussed separately beginning with chapter 4.

I had been studying these ethical principles since the very beginning of my practices in Yoga, and when I arrived in Kashmir in 1988, I begged Lakshmanjoo to tell me more about how these principles were described in the Shaivite philosophy. I was desperately looking for a way to reverse his intention to die. I knew that if anything could catch his interest, it would be conversation about spiritual matters. He had said so many times over the years how much he enjoyed talking to me about these inner aspects of Yoga.

Little by little, the subject attracted his attention, and he began to speak. His voice was very weak and hoarse from nonuse, but he grew stronger every day, and each day he could speak a little longer. We had brought a video camera with us, and he gave us permission to videotape the sessions where we discussed the ethics of Yoga. This book is based on the insights he imparted to me during those precious classes, and I am looking forward to sharing them with you. I have included some of our conversations in this book so you can have the experience of hearing Lakshmanjoo's words directly.

By the time I arrived in Kashmir that summer in 1988, I had been studying Yoga for many years. It all began one summer night in 1952. I went to bed at my usual time, with only the ordinary thoughts that a busy homemaker might have on her mind, and promptly fell asleep. In the middle of the night, I awoke to see a huge column of light at the foot of the bed. It filled the room with its tremendous radiance. I could only remember seeing light such as this when power lines were down after a storm, flashing as they whipped around and then grounded themselves. The light had no shape, but it was rapidly coming closer to me.

In terror, I pulled myself up against the headboard of my bed. I tried to wake my husband, but I found that I could not speak or move my arms or legs. At the time, I was sure that I was not dreaming because I could see the curtains billowing at the window and the branches of the maple tree outside swaying in the breeze. Finally, I gave up and simply watched as the light grew nearer and gradually began to cover me and enter my body. I must have lost consciousness then because the next thing I knew it was morning.

I thought back on the experience and wondered if it had been a dream after all. But as I put my feet on the floor and started to dress, the word "Yoga" sprang into my mind. I brushed my teeth and thought about Yoga. I went to fix breakfast for my family and thought about Yoga. I wondered where this thought had come from. I had never even heard the word before, except at a county fair long ago where a turbaned man claimed that he could tell the future for a small sum.

My family came to breakfast, then the children went off to school, and it seemed like an ordinary day. As my husband lingered over his coffee and paper, I felt that I had to tell him what had happened. He put down his paper and suggested that perhaps I needed a good psychiatrist, and with a few more funny remarks along this line, we dropped the subject.

The thoughts of Yoga did not go away, however. I found that I had entered the brilliant world of the clairvoyant. I sometimes knew what was going to happen before it happened. In dreams, and even in broad daylight, I would see and hear people telling me things about the life I led, the future, and most of all, about Yoga. I began to read and study everything I could find about Yoga, struggling to understand what Yoga was and why it had so suddenly entered my life.

One man appeared in my visions more and more. He was a very large brown man with beautiful eyes. Sometimes in dreams I would see him talking to me earnestly, and I would awake trying to remember what he had said. Then he began to appear to me during the day, usually in my kitchen as I was doing the dishes. At first, I would run from the room in terror. Eventually, though, I became braver and even started to watch for him. He told me that his name was Sivananda, and he began teaching Yoga to me in earnest. One day, he told me to go to the library and look for a particular book, where he said that I would find his address. I thought that I had read every book on Yoga our small library had to offer, but obviously, I had missed one because there it was. I wrote to Sivananda immediately, and our lessons continued, primarily by correspondence, for many years.

In the early 1960s, I finally decided that I had to travel to India to meet Sivananda in person. As I was making preparations, however, he sent word for me not to come. A few months later, I learned that he had died. In my grief, I could not imagine practicing Yoga without his guidance, so I tried desperately to give up my practices and ignore the dreams and visions that suffused my life. From my studies so far, I knew that in advanced practice it becomes necessary to have the guidance of a guru, meaning a teacher who has accepted the responsibility of directing a student's development in Yoga. In the ten years since that first brilliant vision marked the beginning of Yoga in my life, I had never found anyone else in northern Ohio who even practiced Yoga, let alone someone to teach me.

Soon I found that no matter how much I grieved for Sivananda, my life had not changed. Yoga was still there and showed no signs of going away. The deep silence of meditation that I had experienced came slipping back more and more into my mind. So I went back to my daily practices. By now, they had become my essential support.

One day, a year or two later, I received a telephone call from a man named Dr. Kulkarni, who had traveled from India to do research in organic chemistry at Case Western Reserve University in Cleveland. He said that he was in the United States for a year and had met a group of people who were interested in his studies of Yoga. These people had raised enough money to bring his guru, Rama, to the United States for a visit. I asked Dr. Kulkarni how he had heard of me, since, despite my inquiries over the years, I had never come across any group nor talked to anyone who had ever heard of Yoga. He vaguely said that he had just happened to hear about me and asked if I would meet Rama at the airport.

Almost overcome with excitement, I hurried to the airport, stopping just for a moment to pick an armful of lilacs from my garden. (I didn't realize then that the traditional greeting for a guru is flowers.) A beautiful small brown man with clear brown laughing eyes met me. He took my flowers, looked into my eyes, and my heart stopped beating as he said, "Alice, I have come for you."

Rama, the light of my life, became my guru and continued my training. I traveled to India with him in the mid-1960s, when the Indian government had just completed its transition from British rule. I lived in his compound—basically a grass-roofed hut surrounded by a small garden near the Ganges River—for several months of intense study. I traveled with him across India as he lectured and taught.

Before Rama died, in 1972, he told me to go to Kashmir and seek out his friend Lakshmanjoo, who would finish my training. Not really knowing what to expect, I traveled to Kashmir with a group of my students in 1974 (I had been teaching Yoga since 1960). Rama's friends in Kashmir, who kindly helped us with all the preparations for our stay, warned me that Lakshmanjoo probably would not see me since I was an American and a woman, and therefore considered unclean. But Lakshmanjoo sent word that we should come on Sunday, which was his regular day to receive visitors and students.

We had set up our camp on houseboats in a secluded corner of Dal Lake in Srinagar, the capital of Kashmir. The day we went to meet Lakshmanjoo, it was raining heavily. We piled into the little gondola-like boats (called *shikaras*) that were our only form of transportation and set out across the lake in the rain to Lakshmanjoo's compound. We arrived bedraggled, wet, and muddy and stood before the great master in awe. I introduced myself and my students. Lakshmanjoo looked at me long and hard. He said only, "Sing!" So, with quavering voices, we sang some of the Sanskrit devotional songs that Rama had taught us. Much later, Lakshmanjoo told me that his heart had leaped when he saw me, but it would not have been proper for him to show his emotions in front of the Kashmiris who were there.

And so began several years of study with one of the most remarkable men I have ever known. Every summer, I traveled to Kashmir and visited Lakshmanjoo nearly every afternoon, talking about Yoga for hours on end in a little tea house in the midst of his lovely garden. He was a generous and loving teacher who has supported me through all difficult times and, most of all, inspired me to fulfill the expression of Yoga in my life.

I am a full-blown Shaivite now. Through practicing the techniques and attitudes of Kashmir Shaivism described in this book, I have realized a tremendous fulfillment of purpose and strength. I have learned how to use the classical techniques of Yoga (exercises, breathing, and meditation) to form a solid foundation for the experience of joining with my spiritual nature. I have gained great respect for the very different contributions of my physical body and my intellect. Finally, through the diligent practice of Yogic ethics, I have been able to experience the joining of my physical and spiritual bodies, which has given me great strength and has illuminated my life.

In this book, I will show you how to reach for this type of experience in yourself. Everyone knows that Yoga has many physical and mental benefits—such as improved limberness, strength, health, and well-being—but there is so much more to Yoga that is available to the interested student. It is this extra dimension of Yoga that I want to tell you about. This book shows you how you can get to know your spiritual nature and enjoy its blossoming in your life with happiness, strength, and a powerful individuality. It does take some courage to venture into the unknown like this, just as it takes the willingness to follow the impulses of your heart. Rama's motto was "Fearlessness, unity, and bliss," which describes the brave person who seeks meaning in life.

I offer you this book as your guide and teacher, in the hope that it will inspire and support you the way my teachers inspired me. I look forward to sharing this unique journey with you.

A JOURNEY TO YOUR POWERFUL INNER WORLD

Most people associate Yoga with the physical postures and movements that are taught in classes or learned from books. The physical aspect of Yoga, however, is only a small part of the great body of thought and technique that is the tradition of Yoga. In fact, the physical exercises and breathing techniques were originally designed simply to keep the body strong and healthy so that the practitioner could more easily reach for some of the deeper aspects of Yoga.

Most of us eventually find that health and wellbeing are not enough; like most of humanity, we feel a deep longing to find some meaning in life, some reason for being. Many practitioners begin to realize after some time that there is "something else" to be discovered in Yoga that speaks to our universal desire for meaning. While the daily exercises are tuning the physical body into shape, mystical awareness begins to emerge. This happens most often when the ethical practices of Yoga, which are detailed in this book, are combined with the physical routines. Often feelings of inner strength, self-confidence, and inner peace begin to emerge as this other aspect of Yoga starts to reveal itself.

I use the term *mystical awareness* to describe the ability to communicate easily with the inner, deeper, hidden part of yourself, the part that we are less familiar with and that is so rarely observed. Mystical awareness is a powerful gift from the unknown, unseen part of you.

Each person has a slightly different conception of the meaning of words such as *mysticism* and *spirituality*, and I have found that people use such words freely when they are trying to talk about their inner experiences. When I use these terms in class, I can never be sure that my students and I are talking about the same thing because each of us experiences these concepts in our own way. Although it is easy to teach and supervise the routines of exercise and breathing, the inner experiences are always different and difficult to describe.

THE TWO BODIES

I have invented a fantasy game in order to make it easier for me to talk about our subject in a specific way in this book. Instead of relying on words that have such different meanings, I have created a new way of looking at these inner experiences. In this fantasy game, you have not one body to work with, but two: your outer, physical body and a second body that I call the spiritual body. This spiritual body is where the deeper aspects of Yoga reside; this is referred to as the heart of Yoga. The practices described in this book will, I hope, help to make this spiritual body as real to you as your physical body and pave the way for a magnificent union of the two.

Union, in fact, is what the word Yoga means. It is usually understood as a union with yourself. In this book, *union* refers to the joining of your physical and spiritual bodies. This joining

THE SYMBOLISM OF THE HEART IN YOGA

Terms denoting the heart in Sanskrit texts were not meant to be anatomically accurate. Words for "heart" were also frequently used to mean the middle or center or even the bowels, and they represented a variety of emotions, which were said to reside in the heart. References to the heart appear in one of the earliest Indian mystical texts, the *Rig Veda*. Here are a few examples.

"The heart is the organ with which one is able to see what is denied to the physical eye."

"It is the heart which enables a human being to penetrate into deep secrets and mysteries."

"It is in or by the heart that visions are fashioned into words."

"By finding, with or in the heart, the light of higher insight and contact with the transcendent, one becomes an all-seeing rishi [seer]."

This is one example of the richness that awaits when you begin to find yourself. I hope that these lines from the poets of old will inspire you to not only think of your physical heart in your familiar body but also to form a bridge to the heart in your spiritual body that supports and gives power to all you do.

of the two bodies is known in Yogic texts as the creation of the Universal Body. The dynamic state of consciousness that results is described as realization, God consciousness, or, in Sanskrit, *samadhi*. "Realization" means that you now know your whole self; nothing is hidden or unknown. This state brings great peace and strength. When this event takes place, say the Yogic texts, you experience great contentment because there is nothing more to want or learn. The reason for being is answered in full, and you are complete.

Many people believe that this state of realization, or *samadhi*, can be known only by advanced practitioners of Yoga. This is not correct. I believe that anyone can experience glimpses of this state, because the process of getting to know your spiritual body and encouraging it to unite with the physical body is cumulative, and it does not happen all at once. If you use the tools of Yoga that I describe in this book, I have no doubt that, if you want to, you can experience this new type of consciousness yourself.

Let me explain further what I mean by the physical and spiritual bodies. Your physical body is considered to be not only the shell of your skin and what lies inside it, but also your senses, your feelings of "I" and "mine" (also called the feeling of ownership, or the ego), your thoughts, and your intellect. Intellect is the part of you that judges, analyzes, and makes decisions based on your individual perception of the world around you. The word "individual" is important here. The intellect can operate only on the information it receives from your own perception, so its viewpoint is necessarily limited to what you perceive or feel through your senses. The implication in Yoga would be that you cannot truly know what someone else perceives without becoming that other person.

The spiritual body is something else entirely. Most people probably relate the word "spiritual" to their conceptions of God or to feelings that they may have had about the meaning of life or about the universe or perhaps to something pertaining to altered states of consciousness.

As you read this book, I want you to try to drop all your preconceptions and think about the word "spiritual" in a completely different way. As I use the term in this book, spiritual awareness means the ability to open yourself to infinite possibility, where there are no limits to creativity or capability and no restrictions to time, space, mortality, or any other boundary. These are considered to be artificial limits imposed by the physical body's mind and intellect. According to Yoga, the spiritual body can do anything, it knows everything, and it does not die. It is eternal. The physical body works, and the spiritual body feels.

It may help to think of your spiritual body in the shape of an actual body—perhaps just like your physical body, as if you had a Siamese twin attached to you that you did not know about until now. Try to picture this body as the source for all your emotions. We experience our emotions both as beautiful and as somewhat frightening. They seem to be unreliable. We never know when they are going to appear, and sometimes they can be very intrusive in our daily lives.

The physical body reacts without full knowledge of the depth of these emotions. When you experience the protective support of your spiritual body, you can stop the physical reactions that cause discomfort and let the full beauty of emotions from the spiritual body be expressed. In this way, you can learn from your emotions instead of merely reacting to them. When you feel angry, for instance, remember that this feeling is coming from your spiritual body, and realize that it is trying to tell you something that can be used for your strength and protection.

The voice of the spiritual body is intuition. Most people have experienced the clear voice of intuition at some time in their lives, but hardly anyone listens for it consciously. This is because most people rely on their physical bodies for everything and believe that intuition comes from that. They think that they are alone in themselves, with no one and nothing to rely upon except their own abilities and ideas, which, as I said earlier, are limited by their own perceptions because these are produced by the physical body. In this book, you will learn how to listen to intuition and encourage it to speak more often. Intuition is where truth lies. Truth, then, according to Yoga, would lie within the spiritual body.

Imagining a spiritual body is a way to envision the tremendous reservoir of awareness that opens to you when you recognize that there's a great world beyond your own viewpoint. When your physical body tries to figure everything out by itself,

> The subtle Self within
> the living and
> breathing body is
> realized in that pure
> consciousness wherein
> is no duality—that
> consciousness by
> which the heart beats
> and the senses perform
> their office.
> (Mundaka Upanishad)

it has only its own limited understanding to work with; it is ignorant of the enormous power that is available when the two bodies work together. When the physical and spiritual bodies unite in realization (in other words, when they know that each other exists), the experience is similar to a perfect partnership or marriage, in which each partner contributes their individual strengths to form a greater whole.

THE TOOLS OF YOGA

Of course, not everyone practices Yoga in order to reach the ultimate state of realization. Yoga is like a collection of very special tools that you can use to create a wide variety of beautiful things. For instance, practicing just a few Yoga exercises daily can bring you strength, health, limberness, improved circulation and respiration, and relief from stiffness, pain, and depression. Yoga breathing and meditation techniques can help relieve anxiety, insomnia, and stress. These are only a few of the many recognized benefits of Yoga practice.

You do not have to practice Yoga in order to enjoy and benefit from the ideas presented in this book. But if you would like to start, see the Resources section on page 189 for some books and tapes that can help you begin safely. You don't need to commit a great deal of time in order to see these beneficial results. A daily routine of twenty to thirty minutes is quite sufficient at first. Be sure that your routine includes at least a few minutes each of exercise, breathing, and meditation. Yoga should be practiced once during every twenty-four–hour period for best results.

The most important tools of Yoga, the ten ethical principles, can protect and guide you into a happy, productive life. Ethical behavior coaxes your spiritual body into form so you can experience its power. If you practice these principles along

> The power that resides in the heart of consciousness is freedom itself.
> (Abhinavagupta)

with the exercises, breathing, and meditation, you can become more aware of your spiritual body and encourage it to function more openly. Practicing ethics shows you how to realize this inner power source and enjoy it as it blooms in your life, bringing a deeply satisfying awareness of yourself and your world. No longer limited by false perceptions, you enter the limitless universe of self-realization, which is referred to in Yogic texts as "delight, wonder, and astonishment."

This book describes how you can begin your own journey toward discovering the breathtaking power source within you. You will see that the path to this new knowledge is really a simple matter of using new tools. Your spiritual body is already there inside you. As your awareness grows by reading this book and practicing the ideas presented, you will become more conscious of its presence and its supporting power for your physical nature.

HOW TO BEGIN YOUR JOURNEY

In the first three chapters, you will learn how to take the first steps toward this magnificent experience. Chapter 1 further explains the nature of the physical and spiritual bodies according to Yoga and gives you some new ways of visualizing and trying out these new concepts. Chapter 2 describes some of the many ways the experience of realization is approached in Yoga. It is said that the path a student chooses depends on his or her deepest tendencies.

In chapter 3, I will introduce the remainder of the book,

discussing how to begin approaching study and practice of the ethical guidelines of Yoga. Then, chapters 4 through 13 each present a simple outline on how to begin practicing these 10 ethical guidelines. These are the most important chapters because it is impossible to reach the heart of the spiritual body without the practice of ethics. I have tried to talk about each one in a way that shows you the many different levels of approach. For instance, the first ethic, Nonviolence (chapter 4), seems, on the surface, to be very simple to follow: You simply do not cause harm to yourself or others. Yet there are more subtle ways in which violence shows itself, and our discussion will help you explore the many levels of this ethic in a more personal way. Consider these 10 chapters as landscapes that gain more depth each time you visit them. I can assure you of one thing: You will never be bored.

Finally, in chapter 14, I have tried to give you a glimpse into what this union with yourself is really like. I have known two great masters of Yoga who achieved this in full: Rama and Lakshmanjoo. I have experienced it in part myself many times, and those experiences illuminate my life. It is similar to seeing the world in brilliant color after a lifetime of black and white, but more intense.

I wish you all the best as you begin your journey. I have included in this book a few of the experiences my students have had with these techniques. I hope that you will write in care of this publisher and tell me what happens to you during your journey of Yoga.

CHAPTER 1

THE SPIRITUAL BODY: YOUR INNER POWER SOURCE

I n this chapter, I will explain more about my fantasy game of visualizing the physical and spiritual bodies, particularly how they interact and how the practice of ethics facilitates this union. I will also discuss the Yogic meaning of "ego," an important term that is often misunderstood. A correct interpretation of this word is vital in order to practice the ethical principles presented in this book. The correct understanding of ego will encourage the spiritual body to function, thereby opening the door to vast new insights and experiences, such as self-confidence, inner strength, and a new appreciation for yourself.

DESCRIPTION OF THE TWO BODIES

All Yogic literature makes reference to the powerful state of awareness that results when the physical body consciousness joins to the spiritual body consciousness. Some common terms for this experience are self-realization, the Universal Body, or God consciousness, all of which describe a state where all separateness has disappeared and guidance for your life is supplied from within. (I will use these three terms interchangeably in this book.) This state is often described as two lovers joining ecstatically after enduring a long search for each other.

States of being have often been portrayed as God-like forms in artistic representations throughout the world. Such anthropomorphizing serves a valuable purpose because it is difficult to become familiar with something that is unseen. When form is given to these seemingly inexplicable states, one can more easily relate to them—just as, in this book, we are trying to fantasize a form of the inexplicable state of the spiritual body in order to make it more real. You will have two separate bodies to work with: one physical and one spiritual.

WHERE THIS IDEA CAME FROM

When I first began thinking about how to get to know my spiritual nature, I turned to a fantasy exercise to help me discover a form for it. I realized that what I really wanted was to be able to relate to my spirituality in the same way that I would relate to another person. I wanted to see it as a real body, the same as my physical body. I wanted this body of my spiritual nature to be able to speak to me so that I could enjoy its wisdom and revelations, to be so close to me that I would never feel alone again. I wanted this spiritual body to always be there for me, enjoying everything with me. I wanted to enjoy its support in times of need. I wanted the type of closeness experienced by physical twins who are tightly connected in thought and feeling.

If you open yourself fully to the fantasy of the two bodies, you will often be surprised at what occurs. As I continued to

THE UNIVERSAL BODY

One name used for the Universal Body in the Eastern tradition is Shiva. In Yogic literature, Shiva is often given the form of a man, but this form actually represents a state of consciousness. The state of Shiva specifically describes the process of detaching one's consciousness from the limits of the body, whereupon one develops a sense of all-pervasiveness. The sensations of separateness and limitation disappear; there is no longer any difference between the perceiver and the perceived (subject and object). A verse from one of the great books on Kashmir Shaivism comments on this idea, asking rhetorically what the purpose of worship would be once the Highest Reality has been realized.

play, I found that I could visualize the arms and legs of my spiritual body as feelings. I had never considered that emotions such as love, anger, or joy could be pictured as actual parts of a body that reached out to me. Emotions had always seemed mysterious and flighty. I felt buffeted by them constantly, feeling their force but never knowing where they lived or what they looked like. The idea that all emotions could be as substantial as my physical body was a completely new experience for me. As I continued my fantasy over the years, I began to realize that emotions actually can have form and substance. I had always felt their power; they only *seemed* separate and unseen.

This new knowledge showed me how limited my previous outlook had been and opened a door to the freedom of wonderful new experiences. Emotions became as real and factual to me as the chair that I was sitting on or the food that I ate. They were no longer descriptions of how I felt—they began to solidify in form. When I felt love, for instance, I could actually picture love in the room with me.

11

> Without this playing with fantasy, no creative work has ever yet come to birth. The debt we owe to the play of imagination is incalculable.
> (Carl Jung)

The strength of emotional power is usually diluted in our lives; very seldom does it shine clearly as a constant, powerful force in our accomplishments. People who display powerful emotions are often frightening. They seem out of control and unpredictable. Sometimes such people become quite destructive, as when a parent's volatile temper turns to child abuse. It is understandable that control of the emotional nature is encouraged in us from childhood. The tools of Yoga, specifically the practice of ethics, help us to channel the power and strength of emotion that comes through the spiritual body into our physical personality safely and constructively.

The other important realization I had through fantasy about my spiritual body was that it constantly spoke to me through my intuition. I had always heard the voice of intuition in my life, but I never knew where it came from. I know now that it speaks to me directly from my spiritual nature.

As I became more familiar with my spiritual body, I realized that it seems to lie unseen at first, but when I look for it, it takes form in strength and power. It has simply been waiting to show itself. When I encouraged it to express itself, through constant invitation and awareness of its existence, it rewarded me with great insight and constant companionship. Another discovery showed me that the spiritual body emerges in us according to our unique identity. It speaks to us in a language that we can easily understand. No translation from a teacher is necessary in this process because the clear communication comes to ourselves from within ourselves without words.

This process is exactly what Yoga is all about. The tools of Yoga—exercise, breathing, meditation, and ethical behavior—show a person how to build the strength, courage, and determination needed to sustain the emergence of the spiritual body as it joins forces with the physical.

Over time, I have come to know that the spiritual body is the anchoring force in my life. It is the unseen support for my physical body. Actually, the two bodies are interdependent: The physical cannot move without the underlying support of the spiritual, and the spiritual cannot express itself in the world without the form of the physical. Together, they create a complete state of consciousness in which you feel at home in both the seen and the unseen worlds.

THE SYMBOLISM OF THE HERMAPHRODITE

The joining of the two bodies is often represented in mythology by the hermaphrodite—a being half male and half female. The female part of the hermaphrodite represents the physical body, governing action and form, and the male part represents the spiritual body of support and power. They are not two beings, but one. This is the essential premise of Kashmir Shaivism (more fully defined in chapter 2). Both qualities, action (female) and support (male), are necessary for life, and according to Kashmir Shaivism, all life evolves from the con-

THE HERMAPHRODITE

Several Indian sculptures from the fifth century show the image of the god Shiva as a hermaphrodite, half male and half female. In this aspect, the Shiva state represents the union of opposites, showing that the divine is to be comprehended not as separate from the world but inextricably linked to it. The sculptures show us that neither manifest nor unmanifest is more important than the other.

stant, alternating flux of this state of consciousness of one united being.

An easy way to think of this male/female consciousness is to picture waves rippling over the surface of a vast lake. The waves on the surface represent the physical consciousness that is constantly moving, changing, adjusting, and reacting. The waves are actually supported by the deep stillness underneath the surface of the lake, but their movement conceals that stillness.

In the same way, the physical body forgets that it evolves

THE PHYSICAL SELF AS THE STRANGER

The two bodies have been referred to for centuries in Sanskrit terms as *swa-dharma*, which means one's own duty, and *para-dharma*, the duty of what is referred to as someone else. The word *swa-dharma* has two parts: "swa" means self and "dharma" is usually translated as duty, religion, or qualities. The word *para-dharma* also has two parts: "para" means another or stranger, and in this case, "dharma" would mean qualities. Thus *para-dharma* means someone else's qualities, not mine.

The qualities of both bodies are described in many texts. The physical body is described as *para*, or the nonself, of the material world, which includes the physical body and mind. *Swa* describes the spiritual body, consisting of light, power, bliss, fearlessness, and unity. It is immortal, immutable, and all-pervading.

The physical body always feels uncomfortable, as if it does not belong. In other words, the physical personality does not feel at home in the physical body. It is uncomfortable—always looking for relief. The spiritual body does not act that way because it knows that it is already at home. To put it another way, the spiritual body owns the hotel and the stranger (the physical body) is only renting a room.

from the underlying support of the spiritual body. It seems to be living a separate existence, and therefore it always feels a longing to return to that perfect support and calm stillness. People who have not made contact with their spiritual bodies feel this longing constantly.

The spiritual body, on the other hand, never forgets where it comes from—in fact, it never forgets anything. It is not born, nor does it die. It has always been there, fully operational, waiting to be discovered. Encouraging it to emerge is a gift of love to yourself. The trick is to tune in to it, hear it speak, clearly observe its operation, and allow the fragile physical being to rest totally in the protection of its support and tremendous strength. This concept can sometimes feel unsettling because we are most familiar with our physical selves, and so most of us believe that our physical bodies are the strong, dominant partners in our fantasy of the two bodies.

When the spiritual body is first coming into form, through fantasy, you will need to coax it, seduce it, and feed it, because it has had so little attention throughout your life that you may not know how to recognize it, and it may seem reluctant to emerge. But as its form begins to grow and expand in your vision, the idea of physical dominance fades away as the entire relationship becomes balanced and you realize that the two bodies have the potential and desire to become full partners in the state of God consciousness. This is also described in classical texts as fullness of being.

THE ULTIMATE LOVE AFFAIR

The dual-natured consciousness resulting from the joining of the physical and spiritual bodies has been illustrated in poetry and legend throughout the ages as the attraction between a male and a female. They are unable to be apart for even a moment; when they are together, there is total bliss. It is only when they seem to be separate that pain, loneliness, and suffering are experienced. True happiness lies in the realization that they never have been apart and never will be.

When this experience of joining begins to happen—even for a moment at a time—you begin to realize that your physical nature, comprised of body, breath, and mind, is only the tip of the iceberg, a small part of the vast, powerful personality that lies hidden in all human beings. This vast state of consciousness is not usually apparent in the world except in extraordinary circumstances. We sometimes catch a glimpse of it in the superhuman performances of great musicians, dancers, athletes, and others when, for a few moments, they transcend ordinary consciousness and physical limitations, thrilling us with a melodic passion or extraordinary achievement that lifts us out of our everyday existence.

This type of superhuman achievement in Yoga is attained when the person is able to call on the inner spiritual body to join with the outer physical to combine into one force able to accomplish what cannot be done by each half alone. The power that this brings about can be expressed through the thought, "I can be more than I am. I can be all that I have hoped to be—and more." Even more, the pervasive, trapped, discontented feeling of fear that you could never reach the great potential of your dreams disappears as you suddenly know that anything is possible, that any goal can be reached, and that progress is constant.

THE IMPORTANCE OF EGO

The *Bhagavad Gita*, a small section from the classical Indian epic *Mahabharata*, describes universal consciousness in terms of eight qualities.

> Earth, water, fire, air, ether, mind, reason, and also the ego—these constitute my lower [physical] nature. . . . The other than this, by which the whole universe is sus-

tained, know it as my higher [spiritual] nature in the form
of the life principle.

This quotation notes that both bodies, physical and spiritual, are made up of these eight qualities.

In this section, I will focus only on the quality of ego because I believe that using this concept will make it easier for you to make contact with your spiritual body. Because ego is a basic divine substance, it is a property of both bodies. What I call *true* ego is expressed by the spiritual body; *false* ego is expressed by the physical body. Ego is distorted when it is expressed by the physical body—that is why I refer to it as false ego.

An example of this distortion is when you look into a mirror. You know that what you see is only a small part of who you are. You are much more than your physical reflection. In the same way, the false ego sees only a small part of the real you. The picture of your real self will be presented to you by the true perception of your spiritual body. If you can remember these two concepts—false ego and true ego—and notice when they are operating, you will be able to recognize when ego has been distorted by the physical body, and you can begin to enlist the help of your spiritual body with all decisions.

Another reason that this description of the quality of ego is so important is that false ego, which is connected with the physical body, causes the greatest problem in the practice of ethics. I will explain why later in this section.

The ego is a much misunderstood concept in today's world, and it usually has a negative connotation in casual speech. When we say of someone, "He is egotistical," we usually mean that he thinks only of himself. In other words, we equate the term with self-centeredness.

Religion considers ego to be an impediment to spiritual development. You will also find this notion in many translations of Yogic texts, and many Westernized Yoga schools perpetuate the idea that the ego is dangerous, that it is something to be rooted out, given up, or destroyed in order for spiritual progress to take place.

The Shaivite philosophy disagrees with both these viewpoints. As you can see from the *Bhagavad Gita* text quoted at the beginning of this section, ego is considered a divine substance, a basic constituent of both bodies. It can never be destroyed or given up. Ego is credited with supplying the framework for our life support system: It is what gives us the will to stay alive, the impetus to breathe, and the motivation to walk, speak, and perform every other physical action. The ego cannot be destroyed, but it can be observed, and that training in observation is the beginning of making a connection with the spiritual body.

There is a simple game you can play to learn how to differentiate true ego from false ego. All you have to do is notice your emotional reactions and mentally turn them over to your spiritual body. You will find immediate relief. Here's how it works.

Emotional reactions, which often involve some pain or fear, are a fact of daily existence. You can always tell when emotional reactions are threatening your physical body because you will feel uncomfortable. For instance, fear causes uncomfortable feelings of anxiety and muscle tension. The physical nature believes that it must take full responsibility for these reactions and attempt to solve all problems by itself.

This is what I meant when I said that the physical body distorts ego. When faced with a problem, our physical nature acts as if it "owns" the problem. In other words, it does not recognize that help is available from our spiritual nature. In an attempt to relieve its discomfort by itself, the physical body can easily turn to self-destructive behaviors such as alcohol or drugs or neglecting to take care of itself.

Here is a specific example: If you are afraid of a confrontation with a friend, you will feel uncomfortable and anxious even before the confrontation takes place. Perhaps part of your discomfort comes from feeling uncertain about how to handle the situation. Perhaps you cannot sleep well the night before and find yourself unable to eat much because your stomach feels upset.

The moment you notice that feeling of discomfort, you can know that false ego is operating. When you feel that, play my game. Say to yourself, "This is false ego operating. I am uncomfortable. I am going to turn the problem over to my spiritual body for a solution." In other words, you are going to call in an extra support system to deal with the fear. You will find that you register immediate relief. When you invite the spiritual body to help you, you will find that intuition, or your spiritual voice, will suggest a solution to you that can transform an uncomfortable situation into a healing, productive situation. The spiritual body, in fact, heals emotional reaction. The anxiety disappears, the fear leaves, and your body feels calm again. This game can be used in any personal situation where you are faced with an uncomfortable emotional reaction.

This partnership with the spiritual body gives you the extra support you need, a much greater ability to transform any emotion that arises from a potentially self-destructive problem into a constructive solution that not only solves the problem but also gives you new confidence in yourself. As you will see in chapter 4, avoiding self-destructive behavior is an important factor in all ten of the ethical guidelines. Ethical behavior will prove to you that the spiritual body can handle any situation perfectly. Your physical body does not have to carry any burden alone.

But if false ego is such a problem, what can you do about it? The easy formula of Shaivism says that all you have to do is notice when true or false ego is operating. No other change is demanded of you. Simply become aware of it, as in the game I described earlier, by noticing when you feel uncomfortable. According to the Shaivite philosophy, if you can do this, you will be aware when the physical body stands in the way of the true interpretation coming from the spiritual body, and you will have a choice about what to do. You will no longer be trapped by impulse.

ETHICS AND THE FEAR OF DEATH

The freedom of choice is just one of the great benefits of ethical behavior. A most powerful and beautiful experience emerges as you learn to enlist the help of your spiritual body. This is because the spiritual body is always there for you. It exists forever. It does not die. Knowing this will help you overcome the fear of death, which is also a direct product of meditative practice. Meditation allows you to step beyond the restraints of the fragile physical body, which always fears death.

The *Bhagavad Gita* describes this state of mind beautifully. The main characters in the *Gita* are Arjuna, a great warrior trained from birth to regain his rightful kingdom from his unscrupulous cousins in an ultimate battle, and his friend and guru, Krishna, who serves as his charioteer.

As the *Gita* begins, Arjuna is standing in his chariot observing the warriors on both sides of the battlefield. Suddenly, he realizes the tremendous death and destruction that will occur because of this war and is overcome by remorse.

A MEDITATION EXPERIENCE

Once in the early years of my practice of Yoga, I decided to meditate for a few minutes as I was waiting for my family to come home for supper. I sat in a big chair in the living room and quieted myself. Suddenly, I saw myself slip out through my nostrils and hover above my body. I looked down at my body quite peacefully, and eventually slipped back inside. After that experience, I never felt quite the same way about death and loss, because I began to know that I had an existence without my physical body.

Krishna, seeing his grief and fear, speaks the following words, describing the spiritual body as the "soul."

Arjuna, how will anyone who knows this soul to be imperishable, eternal, and free from birth and decay cause anyone to be killed, or kill anyone? As a man discarding worn-out clothes takes other new ones, likewise the embodied soul, casting off worn-out bodies, enters into others which are new.

Weapons cannot cut it nor can fire burn it; water cannot drench it nor can wind make it dry. For this soul is incapable of being cut; it is proof against fire, impervious to water, and undriable as well. This soul is eternal, omnipresent, immovable, constant, and everlasting. This soul is unmanifest; it is unthinkable; and it is spoken of as immutable. Therefore, knowing this as such, you should not grieve.

And Arjuna, even if you regard this soul as constantly taking birth and constantly dying, you should not grieve like this. For in that case, the death of him who is born is certain, and the rebirth of him who is dead is inevitable. It does not, therefore, behoove you to grieve over an inevitable event. Arjuna, all beings were unmanifest before they were born, and will become unmanifest again when they are dead; they are manifest only in the intermediate stage. What occasion, then, for lamentation?

Hardly anyone perceives this soul as marvelous, scarce another likewise speaks thereof as marvelous, and scarce another hears of it as marvelous; while there are some who know it not even on hearing of it. Arjuna, this soul residing in the bodies of all can never be slain; therefore, it does not behoove you to grieve for any being.

So we hear the great guru Krishna instruct his student to march on bravely in his life, totally dependent upon his spiritual

The Self, who is to be realized by the purified mind and the illumed consciousness; whose form is light; whose thoughts are true; who, like the ether, remains pure and unattached; from whom proceed all works, all desires, all odors, all tastes; who pervades all; who is beyond the senses; and in whom there is fullness of joy forever—he is my very Self, dwelling within the lotus of my heart.
(Chandogya Upanishad)

body that will carry him through every battle that is to be fought in this physical world. He asks Arjuna to remember his long practice of ethics, which have prepared him for the battlefield. Arjuna has forgotten this in his terror, and Krishna reminds him that the soul never dies and will carry not only himself through the battle, but everyone else as well.

When ethics are used to prepare the path for the joining of the spiritual and physical bodies, that joining becomes easy. When this happens, you will know that there is no loss in death. In fact, there can be no death. The physical wears out and changes, but the spiritual body is eternal and is never lost. Yoga philosophy says this is the real reason for all practice. Many other benefits are there in plenty, but the big victory is that fear of death is gone forever; death has lost its sting.

DELIGHT, WONDER, AND ASTONISHMENT

Fear of the unknown in ourselves, like fear of death, prevents us from experiencing the full power of our Universal Body. Ethical behavior guides us through fear and allows the unknown in us to come forward as a friend. This, therefore, helps us to open ourselves up to a spontaneous experience that is far beyond our egotistical control or imagination. The result, to use a common phrase in Kashmir Shaivism, is "delight, wonder, and astonishment." The unseen spiritual body then shows its form, a form so dear, so sweet, so absolutely loving that, when it joins the physical, life takes on a shining confidence and power that shows in one's face and demeanor like a mantle of royalty.

And now we are almost ready to begin exploring the ten ethical guidelines in more detail. First, however, I will briefly outline Yoga history and philosophy to give you some background on the many perspectives offered by different schools, including Kashmir Shaivism. This will give you a context in which to place the Yogic tools that I am introducing to you in this book.

CHAPTER 2

MANY ROADS ALL ENDING IN ONE PLACE

T his is not intended to be a scholarly treatise on Yoga philosophy. The subject is so vast that it would be presumptuous of me to try. In addition, I am conscious of the words of my great teachers, Rama and Lakshmanjoo, who cautioned me that the real secrets of Yoga can never be learned—or taught—intellectually. In fact, the intellectual approach can form a wall between you and the powerful, intuitive experience of the spiritual body. That is why, in this book, I have created a fantasy technique that will support a more practical approach to the ethical guidelines of Yoga that can serve you in any circumstance.

THE DIFFERENCE BETWEEN YOGA AND RELIGION

Yoga is not a religion. It is a series of techniques that, when practiced daily, can be used as tools to add meaning and depth to your life, no matter what your religion or background.

We have all grown up with different social backgrounds, religious training, and familial customs, yet Yoga shows how even very simple techniques, practiced in small increments, can bring on the realization that within our outer physical being is a universal spiritual nature. One of the great strengths of Yoga is this premise that there is an underlying spiritual support that is the same in everyone, and there are many paths that lead to its discovery.

No one practices Yoga in exactly the same way as anyone else. Although some of the techniques may appear to be similar, each person's experience is unique. Knowing this fact will smooth away the discordant, abrasive attitude adopted by some practitioners that demands that in order to practice Yoga techniques, you have to think and practice only one way. In Yoga, you are not expected to blindly follow a particular path; you are always guided by your own experience.

Because most Yogic texts were originally written in India, many people sincerely believe that in order to practice Yoga, they must transform themselves into something resembling an Indian. During my long career in Yoga, I have often met people who think that they must change their names, change their dress, and adopt Eastern religious customs. This would be a mistake. Yoga is a very precise discipline that produces very strong individuals who do not have to lean on any external factors in order to identify themselves as practitioners. Yoga will not interfere with your personal religious faith. In fact, many students say that Yoga strengthens their personal beliefs by providing a strong underpinning of confidence, self-awareness, and well-being.

Many dictionaries mistakenly define Yoga as an offshoot of the Hindu religion. Historical evidence of Yoga practice actually predates Hinduism by many centuries. Unlike religion, Yoga does not advocate rituals or creeds. Also, as any serious practitioner will tell you, when one attempts to approach the summit in Yoga practice, one must go on alone, dependent on

THE QUESTION OF CULTS

Not everyone is comfortable with the self-motivation that is at the heart of Yoga. People who feel the need for religious rules and beliefs are easy prey for charismatic leaders who seem to offer easy answers to life's problems. Many people want someone else to tell them what to do, how to live, and how to be happy, and they often believe that a leader with a strong personality will be a type of savior. This kind of relationship has no place in Yoga. A true teacher realizes that your desires must be answered by you, and it is the teacher's responsibility to point that out and show you how to do it. The teacher then provides the support and encouragement you need during your search.

The jewel of Yoga is that if you can find the courage to face that journey into yourself, you become your own savior. You have the ability to become strong, content, and fulfilled without depending on something or someone outside yourself. The spiritual body that you possess contains all the knowledge that you will need to reach the highest pinnacle of your life. Yoga techniques and philosophy form a bridge to finding yourself within yourself.

only the spiritual body that is now coming into view.

Throughout this book, I do mention terms that may have religious connotations for you, such as "God," "God consciousness," and "spiritual." No one can really know what the supreme consciousness is like. Since any words become inadequate in the face of this immense concept, I decided to use terms that will be familiar to most people. The best way to read these words is to give them a personal reference that means something to you.

People often ask about the meaning of the huge pantheon of gods and goddesses pictured in the art of the Eastern world.

These images are often misunderstood in the West. Actually, these many different forms are used to represent the many emotional personalities of the great state called God consciousness or the Universal Body. They are the moods and expressions of one being, the supreme force that is the source and support for all creation.

These various images represent powerful emotional forces in this world that have no physical form. Consider love, for instance. Everyone has heard about love, and some people believe that they can describe it. A great deal of money is spent in the corporate world to convince people that love can be attained through the right cosmetics, beer, greeting cards, perfumes, and other products. Although we are all influenced by these efforts, we know that, in reality, love cannot be packaged. Love has no form; it remains unseen, though it can be felt. The same can be said of any emotion. It can be felt, but it cannot be packaged.

Eastern art pretends that these unseen emotions can take form, and because of the enormous respect shown to emotions in this context, they are referred to in divine terms. These gods have been given a humanlike form in order to make them easier to relate to. They portray the emotions of the spiritual body in their purest, most subtle form and express themselves through the physical body.

Let's return to the example of love. I believe that love can be experienced in its full depth only by quieting the physical body and inviting the clear expression of love to flow through you from the spiritual body. The joint efforts of your outer (physical) and inner (spiritual) natures are needed to bring this experience of love to its ultimate expression. By combining the forces of the physical and spiritual bodies in this way, you can experience the full expression and subtlety of not just love but all emotions.

The Shaivite philosophy says that this entire divine pantheon of emotions lies within you, waiting for you to call them forth in all their beauty and strength. These forms of gods and goddesses, then, simply represent parts of you. They are what you have always been but have been unable to recognize. They are a picture of your spiritual body in all its power.

HOW YOGA BEGAN

The short answer is, nobody knows. The origins of Yoga certainly predate written history. Archaeologists have found seals with carvings of people in Yoga positions that date back more than 5,000 years.

Even after the advent of writing, Yoga was usually transmitted by word of mouth, handed down from teacher to student. Only a few texts on Yoga remain from that early period, written in a sort of enigmatic code of aphoristic statements that have meaning only to the serious student of mystical experience. Of course, these documents have been extensively commented on by various prominent scholars.

I was fortunate in having two powerful teachers who introduced me to these great writings. Lakshmanjoo was well-known for his translations of the writings of a great teacher named Abhinavagupta, who lived in the tenth century in Kashmir and was the author of a brilliant commentary on Kashmir Shaivism. Rama taught me the principles of Vedantic thought, a system of Yoga philosophy that teaches realization of the self through a systematic transformation of the five sheaths that hide the true self in three states of consciousness (as shown below).

State of Consciousness	Sheath
The waking state	(1) the physical body and the material world
The dream state	(2) the "vital forces" such as breath, (3) the mind, and (4) the faculty of understanding
The deep sleep state	(5) "bliss"

The Vedantist considers the entire material world, as expressed in these five sheaths, to be an illusion that cannot last, and so the practitioner attempts to refuse its entrancements. In contrast to Kashmir Shaivism, an inclusive philosophy, Vedanta is exclusive. The practitioner constantly moves away from attachment to the world by saying, "Not this, not that"—in other words, "I am not a mother. I am not a father. I am not a child. I am not this ego. I am not this mind"—and so on until he or she is left with the only thing that is real, lasting, and unchanging: the true self.

CLASSICAL YOGA
AND PATANJALI

One of the great classical Yogic texts was written by the scholar Patanjali, who lived sometime between the third century B.C. and the third century A.D. He made a great contribution by observing the many different Yoga techniques and theories that people were practicing at the time and organizing them into a coherent form in his *Yoga Sutras*.

The system that is described as Classical Yoga has eight parts. These eight parts represent eight stages of consciousness, or states of awareness, that reside in both the physical and spiritual bodies. Lakshmanjoo called these eight steps limbs and taught me the importance of practicing them simultaneously rather than one by one.

The Sanskrit names for the eight limbs (or centers of consciousness), along with their usual English translations, are *yama* (restraint), *niyama* (observance), *asana* (posture), *pranayama* (breath technique), *pratyahara* (withdrawal of the mind from the senses), *dharana* (concentration), *dhyana* (meditation), and *samadhi* (absorption).

The words *yama* and *niyama* describe the ten ethical guidelines that I am presenting in this book in chapters 4 through 13. The next two, *asana* and *pranayama*, are the exercises and

FOUR TYPES OF STUDENTS

The *Bhagavad Gita* describes four types of students who come to Yoga: the sufferer, the seeker for worldly goods, the seeker for knowledge, and the man of wisdom. In other words, most people are drawn to Yoga by an underlying need or desire. That need may be an unresolved hurt, a strategy for health and success, or a drive for completeness. Even if you are not a student of Yoga, you can probably see how your deepest desires determine the course of your life and the efforts you make to obtain those desires.

As a teacher, I see all types of students in my classes, and usually, they practice Yoga until their underlying needs are met, then they stop. Not everyone can have the same goals or move toward them at the same pace. The tools of Yoga can be used as long as they are needed. If you are lucky enough to have a teacher who can show you how to practice correctly, anything is possible.

breathing techniques that most people are taught in Yoga classes in the West. *Pratyahara* is the beginning stage of meditation, where you learn to turn your attention from the outside world to the internal. *Dharana*, *dhyana*, and *samadhi* are three stages of meditation, where the student learns to focus on one point for longer and longer periods of time until, in the final stage, the student attains the ability to remain in that focused state for as long as he or she wishes and to move in and out of that state at will.

TYPES OF YOGA

There are more than 100 different schools of Yoga. Following are some of the most well-known ones.

Hatha Yoga: The physical movements and postures, plus

breathing techniques. This is what most people associate with Yoga practice.

Raja Yoga: Called the royal road because it incorporates exercise and breathing practice with meditation and study, producing a well-rounded individual.

Jnana Yoga: The path of wisdom; considered to be the most difficult path.

Bhakti Yoga: The practice of extreme devotion in one-pointed concentration upon one's concept of God.

Karma Yoga: All movement and all work is done with the mind centered on God.

Tantra Yoga: A way of showing the unseen consciousness in form through specific words, diagrams, and movements. One diagram used to show the joining of the physical and spiritual bodies is of two triangles superimposed upon one another. The downward-pointing triangle represents the physical body, or the female aspect of work, action, and movement, while the upward-pointing triangle represents the spiritual body, or the male aspect of support, energy, and vastness.

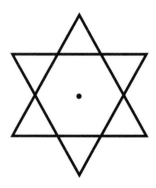

Yoga is unique in that, in the beginning, each person experiences something different, although as practices progress, everyone ends up at the same ultimate point. The different types of Yoga briefly outlined above are broad categories only. Most practitioners choose from among them according to their needs, desires, and of course, what they have been taught.

As already mentioned, I practice Kashmir Shaivism, which is a philosophy that intrigued me from the very beginning of my study of Yoga. Both my teachers instructed me in this school, which holds that everything in the universe is both male and female. Some words that describe the male principle are heat, dryness, energy, mind, and potentiality. The female principle can be described in terms such as cold, wetness, movement, and form.

Many Yogic philosophies recognize only the male principle, saying that the female aspect—that is, the manifest world—is unreal. That is why you often see pictures of ascetics attempting to negate their bodies through suffering and self-denial. They are attempting to prove to themselves that the world, or the female aspect, is not important. This external austerity, or an outward practice for show, is a clear picture of false ego. In this book, I am attempting to describe the opposite: an internal observance in which practice is done within yourself, for yourself alone.

Kashmir Shaivism recognizes that the male and female principles are equal partners, that they are interdependent and cannot be separated. They are, in fact, one thing. The feeling of attraction between them creates the immense complexity of the universe that we enjoy and celebrate.

In summary, Kashmir Shaivism is an approach that is inclusive, rather than exclusive. The entire universe and everything in it is considered divine and composed of this male/female principle, the two aspects of which are always longing for union with each other. This picture of the universe is represented in us by the image of two bodies: spiritual and physical. Both are equally powerful, and both are necessary for a complete world—and a complete individual. Kashmir Shaivism observes the total world as part of yourself, and none of it is to be rejected. You are taught to observe and learn from everything. In this way, you are able to make a choice about how to live your life.

CHAPTER 3

INTRODUCTION TO THE TEN ETHICAL PRINCIPLES OF YOGA

As discussed, Classical Yoga is comprised of eight parts, called limbs (see page 30). Most classes in Yoga in the Western world begin with steps three, four, and five—physical exercises, breathing techniques, and beginning meditation techniques. These aspects of Yoga are perfect for those wishing to use Yoga for such goals as flexibility, improved sports performance, relief from anxiety and stress, and improved health. All these are quite valid reasons for practicing Yoga and provide a healthy way to get more out of life.

Some people, however, are reaching for something more. They are becoming aware that life has a much greater source of awareness, and they feel a need to get to know the huge spiritual nature that lies within all of us. This goal requires conscientious attention to the system of Yogic ethics. It is interesting to note that in traditional Yoga practice in India many years ago, a student was required to be firmly established in these ethical practices even before obtaining instruction in the physical exercises, breathing, and meditation techniques.

Remember that in this book, I am using the word "ethics" differently from the social or religious connotations that you may be familiar with, in which ethics are used primarily as a way of relating to the community outside yourself. In Yoga, ethics are practiced in order to develop a relationship with your inner self.

The Sanskrit term *yama* literally means "restraint," and *niyama* means "not restraint" or observance. I have decided to use the English word "ethics" to encompass all ten guidelines because it most clearly depicts the connection between behavior and feeling—in other words, the connection between the physical and spiritual bodies.

Every chapter includes the Sanskrit name of each ethic as well as its most common English translation. I have included these Sanskrit terms because their meanings are complex and cannot be conveyed by a single English translation. As you read and sound out the word phonetically in your mind, there is a deeper, different effect than reading it in English translation. Lakshmanjoo often pointed out that words and sentences were the coarsest form of communication.

When I lived in the jungle with Rama, he used to give me books about Yoga written in Sanskrit, German, and other languages that I hadn't the faintest idea how to read. When I questioned him, he explained that I should look at them anyway, because the information they contained would enter my unconscious and become available to me when I needed it. This type of practice obviously takes a great deal of faith.

AEROBICS FOR YOUR SPIRITUAL HEART

In the following ten chapters, you will learn how to begin making the ethical powers of Yoga a part of your daily life and thought. Think of it as aerobics for your spiritual heart. Just like exercise for your physical body, it works best if you do a little every day.

Each chapter begins with a general definition of the ethic and a brief description of how I will approach it from the viewpoint of Kashmir Shaivism. Then I offer suggestions for how to start practicing the ethic right now. The final sections of each chapter present some discussions about the results gained from practicing this ethic.

Lakshmanjoo told me that, in the same way that a baby's limbs grow all at once rather than one by one, the ten ethics of Yoga all need to be developed simultaneously. This means that even when you are concentrating upon one ethic at a time, you should try to maintain awareness of the other nine principles in the background.

Remember that you are not expected to reach perfection, but are simply doing this to increase your awareness. Try this technique that has worked well for me: Post the list of ten Yogic ethics on your refrigerator, in the bathroom, or any other place in your home where you will see it a few times a day. At the end of the day, take a few moments to think about how you have become aware of each one. Some people have found it helpful to keep a journal of their experiences.

You can also try a simple technique that many of my students have found helpful: Put a small piece of tape or an adhesive bandage on the inside of your wrist and make a small mark whenever you become aware of a success or failure in your ethical practice throughout the day. This technique not only gives you a tangible, visual result but also increases your awareness because you are making a physical mark to record a mental process. (If you are worried that people in your home or work environment may look askance at tape on your wrist, you can place the tape on a notebook, a calendar, or some other place where you will see it often. But the technique works best when you wear the tape.)

If you are like most people, you will probably notice that you are not able to practice each ethic perfectly each day.

> The conscious mind allows itself to be trained like a parrot, but the unconscious does not—which is why Saint Augustine thanked God for not making him responsible for his dreams.
> (Carl Jung)

Your own judgment of your observance of ethics in daily life will determine what perfection means to you. As you repeat these exercises daily, your awareness will constantly increase. If the joyous day comes when you have been aware of practicing all ten ethics in one day, you can congratulate yourself. It is a wonderful feeling.

Try not to feel discouraged if it seems like an impossible task; look upon it as a heroic journey that will lead you to unimaginable riches. No effort is in vain. In all the books I have read on Yoga, the assurance is made that every single step you take toward the formation of the Universal Body can never be lost. The *Bhagavad Gita* makes this promise. In it, Arjuna, the great warrior, turns to Krishna, his friend and teacher, and asks: "Krishna, he whose mind is diverted from Yoga, failing to reach perfection, what fate does he meet with? . . . Does he not perish like the torn cloud, deprived of both God realization and worldly enjoyment?"

Krishna replies: "Dear Arjuna, there is no fall for him either here nor hereafter. For none who works for God realization meets with an evil destiny. He who has fallen from Yoga, having attained the higher worlds, . . . takes birth in the house of pious and wealthy men. Or, if he has developed dispassion, he may be born into the family of enlightened Yogis. . . . There he regains the understanding of his previous births, and through that, he strives, with greater vigor than before, for perfection."

Many people worry that they may fail. To me, the only definition of failure is refusing to face the challenge of whatever lies in front of you. When Arjuna became fearful and told

A PERSONAL EXPERIENCE
WITH ETHICS

A student wrote this wonderful letter about his experiment with ethical behavior.

I discovered that a lot of the restraint I had put upon myself was meaningless and had nothing to do with ethics. So I gave up my ethics in an experiment for forty-eight hours. I kept up all my other Yoga practices, but I was as aggressive as I felt like and let all sexual thoughts occur. During those two days, it really felt like letting air out of a balloon. All my pressure went away and my life seemed to slow down.

Then I went back to my ethical practices with a new awareness of their meaning for me. Who knows if I am doing them perfectly, but I am paying attention and I am trying to do my best. If I screw up, that's understandable. And then I start again. Right?

So there are many things going on that I didn't notice. But after I stopped and then started again, I found out that all this neat stuff happened. I won the second race of the season. Somebody gave me tickets to a concert. Somebody else gave me a discount rental on a boat. Yesterday, my best friend walked in, wanted to buy a car, and then bought it from me. I've had people falling all over themselves to buy cars from me this week. My kids won their basketball games, the dog's in heat, my head is full, and—I hesitate to use the term, but I feel high. This may sound silly, but I feel like I'm full inside. And of course, that doesn't surprise me. My wife has told me that I'm full of things more than once. . . .

Krishna, "I don't want to fight" (see page 20), he was moving toward failure. His teacher urged him to the fight, telling him that although he may fail, failure has only to do with whether or not he makes the attempt. It is similar to learning to play the piano; you cannot expect to play as expertly as Rubinstein in a week, a month, or even a year. It takes the experience of many failures to learn how to succeed. Succeeding means constant observation of yourself in all circumstances.

UNDERSTANDING
VERSUS REALIZATION

If you are like most people and enjoy answers, conclusions, and reasons, you may find yourself struggling to grasp many of the more subtle points in our discussions of the ethics. This book is not a morality tale where you will get "rules to live by." Each chapter will challenge you to learn in a new way as your spiritual body begins to take form and express itself.

The problem with intellectual understanding is best illustrated by a conversation I had with Lakshmanjoo when we were talking about Nonviolence, the first ethic described in this book.

> ALICE: You have said that everything is God. If that is so, then what makes an action either violent or nonviolent?
> LAKSHMANJOO: That is to be realized. When realization is there, then whatever you do is fine. It is for you to realize yourself.
> ALICE: The idea that "everything is God" is easy to say, but it's very hard to understand.
> LAKSHMANJOO: Not to understand—to realize. They are different. One is intellectual, the other is emotional. To realize is to feel the truth.

Lakshmanjoo was pointing out to me that asking to understand is an intellectual demand and that realization is a totally

THE LANGUAGE OF THE HEART

The *Bhagavad Gita* opens as the warrior Arjuna asks his friend and guru, Krishna, to place his chariot between two armies so he can see who is about to take part in the battle. Arjuna sees in his own and the opposing armies all his relatives and friends, and even his old teacher, a person of great reverence. He is suddenly overcome with weakness and fear about the coming battle. He throws himself down in the bottom of his chariot and refuses to fight.

Many great teachers have said that the battle can be seen to stand for the battle among all the disparate parts of an individual—mind, intellect, senses, ego, and so on—in trying to become a whole, united, powerful being. The war is pictured as a battle with the false ego. All interpretations try to illustrate how it is intuition, not intellectual understanding, that supplies the correct approach to these difficult concepts.

Arjuna's distress showed that the ramifications of this important battle went far beyond his limited perception. He couldn't understand what was going on, and he was overcome by his emotions. He had to drop his false egotistical personality and depend totally on the clear voice of the spiritual body, which, in this case, was emanating from his guru. Because he and his guru both were sustained by the same spiritual body, and because Arjuna had the strength to stop objecting long enough to listen to what was being said and let it speak to his spiritual self, realization came quickly. As Rama said once in a lecture on the *Gita*, "Lord Krishna's talk was in the language of the heart. And the language of the heart is known by every human being wherever he may live."

different experience. My naive statement about understanding would apply to the physical body, the residence of the intellect. Realization, on the other hand, has to do with the truth, which resides in the spiritual body.

The brilliant voice of intuition describes the realization that comes like a gift from the spiritual body. This voice of intuition can replace the repetitive, closed-circuit conversations of your physical self talking to yourself inside your head. The truth of all situations will speak from your heart.

Intellectual understanding is based on separateness because it demands proof and because it cannot see outside its own limits. Realization of the spiritual nature needs no proof and has no limits. Lakshmanjoo pointed out this clear difference when he corrected my use of the word "understand." Our conversation continued.

> ALICE: Many people think that realization is a religious phrase.
>
> LAKSHMANJOO: No, it's not a saying; it is to become the state of realization.
>
> ALICE: It's a state of being?
>
> LAKSHMANJOO: Being or becoming, these are the two things. Being is already there in the physical. Becoming lies in the spiritual.

Realization means awareness of the limitless possibilities expressed in the word "becoming." The potential is already there in your heart. To reach that state of becoming, you have to provide the path for the avenue of expression that will allow your spiritual body to join with your physical body in the most harmonious and spontaneous way, as if you were planting a garden with no preconception of what will bloom.

My purpose in bringing this distinction to your attention is to convince you that it does not matter if you do not understand all the points of each ethic that I will be discussing. What matters is that you simply observe, listen, and then let your spiritual body take care of absorbing the message. It takes a type of humility to drop the demand for intellectual mastery, but I can tell you that when you succeed, the result is a delightful new awareness.

THE RESULT OF PRACTICING YOGIC ETHICS

The primary benefit of practicing these ten ethical disciplines, as stated previously, is to facilitate the joining of the physical and spiritual bodies. Another result is a shining phenomenon that I call peripheral awareness. Someone with this quality has a mature thought process that transcends the circular self-talk that goes on in our heads most of the time. It encompasses a much wider environment. People with peripheral awareness can concentrate on whatever job is at hand and still be aware of everything else that is going on in the room. They can handle multitudinous detail without stress.

In addition, the texts of Yoga state a specific result, called a power, that is obtained from the perfect practice of each ethic. For example, the result of practicing Nonstealing is that "all wealth comes to you." According to this idea, ethics can be considered a very practical undertaking.

People spend most of their lives trying to achieve such goals, but their mistake is thinking that their goals are outside themselves. Yoga teaches you to reach within yourself for your goals. Everything you could ever want is there. This is not a narcissistic attitude of self-involvement. On the contrary, it is a powerful practice that not only benefits you but also, eventually, greatly affects everything and everyone around you. As the old blues song goes, "God bless the child that's got his own." You realize that everything you want lies within yourself.

As you think about the results of these practices, try to transform your attitude from one of "getting" to one of "giving." Once in Kashmir I was with Lakshmanjoo when a student came to him and asked, "How can I get more devotion?" I realized immediately that the question should have been "How can I *give* more devotion?" In other words, devotion is not a selfish act. In practicing the ethics of Yoga, one only gives, one never demands—it is not a bargaining situation. With simple humility, you give your spiritual body a welcoming entrance into the physical in order for it to do its work. By doing so, you give yourself a priceless gift that enriches your life unimaginably.

Rama used to tell me: "You give a glass of milk and you get back a cow." It takes only a little practice to enjoy the great benefits of these marvelous tools of Yoga.

CHAPTER 4

ETHIC #1
NONVIOLENCE

Don't Harm Yourself

The Sanskrit name for this first ethic is *Ahimsa*, which is usually translated as nonviolence. Most people are aware that Nonviolence is associated with Yoga, and practice begins by concentrating on not harming yourself.

Nonviolence is listed as the first of the ten ethics because the practice of the other nine depends on it. For example, as you're trying to practice Truthfulness (ethic #2), you will realize that lying to yourself is a form of causing harm to yourself. In the same way, stealing from yourself or others (ethic #3) is a form of harming yourself. So you can see that as you become more aware of this ethic of Nonviolence, you will have a head start on practicing all the other ethics as well.

Harming ourselves most often manifests as self-destructive behavior. Some common examples of self-destructive behavior that we engage in often—many times unconsciously—are when we overeat; overindulge in substances such as alcohol, caffeine, or sugar;

neglect wearing a seat belt while driving; become stressed by overwork; and fail to get enough rest. You can probably think of several other examples.

Do not misunderstand me and think that I will be lecturing you about reforming your lifestyle. On the contrary, as a Yoga teacher, my job is to help you become more aware of what you do and why you do it so you can make a choice. If you consciously practice Nonviolence, for instance, you will not feel the need to overindulge in something like alcohol because you know that it would harm your body and reduce your capacity for safety. Similarly, when you practice this ethic, you gain great regard for the wonderful qualities of your mind and realize that using mind-destroying drugs would cause violence to yourself.

I have found that most self-destructive behavior is caused by feelings of guilt or fear: For instance, when you're stressed, you might lash out at co-workers or family, but afterward, you might feel guilty and berate yourself for losing your temper. Practicing Nonviolence is a way to reduce those feelings of guilt. At the same time, as the need to lash out leaves you, you will be less afraid of retaliation.

In this new awareness of what causes you harm, you must also include so-called passive-aggression, or violence caused by refusing to act, the results of which are often as harmful to you as overt violence. A newly married woman I knew many years ago neglected to remind her husband that her birthday was approaching, thinking to herself, "If he loves me, he will remember on his own." When the day came and she began receiving congratulations from friends, he was greatly embarrassed and humiliated because he had forgotten, and her feelings were terribly hurt. Her choice not to act therefore caused harm to both of them.

The practice of this ethic of Nonviolence teaches you how to protect yourself from your own self-destructive behaviors.

AN EXPERIENCE
WITH NONVIOLENCE

This letter from a student shows how Nonviolence helps reduce self-destructive attitudes.

I had been really focusing on Nonviolence when I started using your "I Love You" Meditation Technique [see Resources on page 189]. I began to feel saturated with a wonderful feeling, as if something was filling all the fissures in my psyche. It was more than a feeling of good self-esteem; it was as if I had uncovered an underground foundation of support that was being reinforced or called into awareness.

Throughout the next week or so, I also noticed a new awareness of my own sense of vulnerability—a feeling from which I've always felt that I had to protect myself. It's almost as if as a child, I made a vow never to allow myself to become really vulnerable. I know that I may not have consciously made such a choice, but as I look back on my life, that concept seems ever-present.

The "I Love You" technique combined with my work on Nonviolence provided me with a feeling of being loved that is not contingent on approval or judgment or external to myself. I don't have much experience with experiencing this feeling at all, especially over an extended period of time. But thus far, I do feel quite different. It doesn't seem to depend on someone else loving or liking me.

I feel something underneath the psychological processes of simply improving my self-esteem that will really support me no matter what. There is an acceptance of myself as I am.

Eventually, your practice will begin to affect others in the world. In fact, Yogic texts say that when a nonviolent person is present, the violence in the immediate environment must subside. I must add that this happens only when the person reaches a great mastery of the practice. Yoga states, however, that even in the beginning of the practice of Nonviolence, by not harming yourself, you are, in a way, automatically not harming others, because all life is considered to come from the same divine source.

The result of this constant attention to not harming yourself is that you eventually become free from a great many upsets that are caused by fear and guilt. If you do not fear retaliation or confrontation, and if, during the course of the day, you manage to reduce your self-destructive behavior even a little, you can go to bed at night thinking that you have done your best, and you can sleep well.

HOW TO BEGIN PRACTICING NONVIOLENCE

Observe uncomfortable feelings. In my experience, feelings of discomfort usually signal that something is hurting you (whether inside or outside). As soon as you notice these feelings, ask yourself whether you are harming yourself in some way. It may take some time before the reasons for your discomfort reveal themselves, especially if you are not used to acknowledging your feelings. If you indeed discover that you are being self-destructive in some way, try the two fantasy exercises below to help you get back on track.

Visualize violent feelings as a separate being. Through practicing this fantasy exercise, you will feel disconnected from those feelings and can avoid harm that would be caused by saying or doing something violent. Pretend, for instance, that someone has said something very hurtful to you and you feel anger toward that person. You would really like to "get back" somehow. You cannot shake that feeling, and it is making you uncomfortable. Pretend that your violent feelings have a body and a shape, as if they were a person standing next to you. To take revenge upon the person who maliciously hurt you, you would have to order this personification of violence to act in your name according to your specifications. You would be asking violence to operate for your own use. You would be making a slave of violence.

Remember, according to our premise in this book, you cannot own violence, or any other emotion. If you think that you can, you are operating from false ego. Violence exists without you. You are simply an observer. Training in the ethic of Nonviolence helps you observe violence in this new way. In turn, seeing violence as separate from you makes it easy to choose your behavior, and therefore accept responsibility for it.

Use fantasy beforehand to protect yourself. This is an exercise that is especially helpful if you know that you are heading into a situation that may become destructive. Suppose that you need to have a meeting with a subordinate about that person's faulty work on a project. The person has been difficult to deal with in the past, and you are dreading the meeting. You do not want to harm yourself by becoming stressed and ill prior to the meeting, and if the person reacts angrily to you, you want to try to explain the truth of the situation without causing harm either to the other person or to yourself.

To help yourself through such situations, practice this exercise when you have a few minutes alone. Sit quietly, close your eyes, and relax your body and breath. Then, imagine that you are standing at the end of a long hallway. There are doors on either side of the hall, and one of them is labeled "Meeting with [person's name]." Before you do anything else, notice that there is a suit of armor hanging on a hook next to you. Visualize all its various shapes and colors and fastenings as you would like them to be. Put on the armor carefully, piece by piece, making sure that your entire body is protected. Buckle on your sword, feeling its weight and power.

You are now ready to face the meeting in your fantasy.

Walk to the door that opens to your meeting, open the door, and stand there, observing what is in the room. You do not have to do anything or go any farther unless you want to. If the person you are meeting is in the room, observe what he or she does and says. If you want to respond, do so, always remembering that you are completely protected. When you have had enough, close the door, walk back to the end of the hall, remove your armor, and slowly bring yourself back to your everyday surroundings. This fantasy exercise can help you practice and prepare for any difficult situations that you have to face.

Protect yourself from illness. Life is precious. I like to think of the things I do to take care of myself as feeling or tasting sweet because I love their effects. For instance, I take vitamins every day. I do not like the taste of vitamins, but I like what they do for me. So vitamins become sweet to me. I have transformed my reaction to them. I have chosen to make them sweet. In the same way, I do not like the constriction of wearing a seat belt in the car, but I like knowing that I am protected from serious injury by wearing it, so wearing it then becomes sweet to me.

Try this test in every area of your life. Does the food you eat give you a sweet feeling or does it make you uncomfortable? Remember that discomfort is the most obvious sign that you are doing something that may be harmful to you or someone else. Observe your relationships. Are they full of demands and disappointments that make you feel uncomfortable, or are they fulfilling and enjoyable?

Watch your inner conversation. Do you find yourself constantly calling yourself a failure, ugly, incompetent, miserable, ill, and so on? Perpetuating negative attitudes about yourself is clearly a violent action. Always return to observation and feeling. "What am I doing? Does it feel sweet or does it feel uncomfortable and painful?" If there is discomfort, you can be sure that you are harming yourself in some way.

This practice brings great power, because increasing your observation of your feelings and reactions paves the way for the emergence of the spiritual body and its expression. Usually the physical body acts as a policeman to the spiritual body, which has a natural inclination to be free. Continually restraining its freedom is a form of violence toward you and your spiritual self. When you remove this restraint, the result is delight, wonder, and astonishment.

NONVIOLENCE AND FOOD

The Shaivite philosophy believes that it is not only the food itself but your desire for food that supports your body. This idea addresses a very primitive feeling that arises in all living things when encountering another being: Am I going to eat it or is it going to eat me? This is obviously a feeling loaded with fear because no living thing wants to be killed and eaten.

I have already talked about how self-destructive behavior manifests in overindulgence or in ingesting too much of a substance that can harm you, such as alcohol or drugs. Moderation in food and drink is a way to practice nonviolence, because the body is then able to use what it needs without becoming stressed having to defend itself against the onslaught of overindulgence. When you practice Nonviolence, you learn to choose to eat what is protective and helpful, protecting yourself from the self-destructive behaviors concerning food that we have discussed previously.

Yoga says that different foods have different qualities inherent in them. You are probably already aware of how certain substances, such as sugar and caffeine, affect your moods. In the *Bhagavad Gita*, there is a clear division of food into three main types according to how they affect a person. These three categories correspond to the three *gunas*, tendencies or qualities of nature, which are found in everything in the world in varying amounts.

1. *Sattwa guna* describes attributes of calmness, purity, and balance. Sattwic food, according to the *Gita*, promotes longevity, intelligence, strength, health, happiness, and delight. It is sweet, not too spicy, nourishing, and good-tast-

ing. In other words, *sattwic* food promotes both physical and emotional health. Some examples of sattwic food would be fruits, vegetables, milk, and whole grains.

2. The attributes of the second category, *rajas guna*, are activity, passion, and restlessness. *Rajasic* food is bitter, acidic, salty, spicy, dry, and pungent. It excites the body's systems. Some examples of rajasic food are hot spices and extremely salty foods.

3. The third quality of nature is the *tamas guna*, which is characterized by sleep, ignorance, dullness, and inertia. *Tamasic* food is that which is nonnutritive, rotten, leftover, or stale. It contributes to listlessness, dullness of mind, and depression. Some examples are "empty-calorie" foods such as diet colas, artificial foods, and probably anything that has been sitting in your refrigerator for more than a week. Meat is considered a *tamasic* food because it is dead and, therefore, inert.

All the qualities described in the *gunas* about food describe attributes of the physical body, which is constantly changing. The spiritual body is the resting place of the feelings that foods inspire in you.

These three *gunas* actually reside in every food, though each food carries a predominance of one of the three qualities. Yoga says that these qualities, such as sweetness, passion, or dullness, actually reside in the food and are then expressed in your body. Food is used as the vehicle for expression of feeling that comes from the spiritual body. A Yogi, for instance, would say that the quality of sweetness "lives" in fruit and is transferred to your body when you eat it, expressing itself in you as a feeling of sweetness. Likewise, the quality of excitement lives in spices, so when you eat spicy foods, the quality of excitement expresses itself in you.

In the same way, it is felt that violence lives in meat. This concept is discussed in ancient Yogic texts, where the eating of meat is compared to eating the quality of violence itself. By killing in order to eat, you have moved into that primitive feeling of fear and aggression, and the violence that lives in the meat expresses itself through you. This is why a vegetarian diet is usually associated with Yoga and the practice of Nonviolence.

You certainly do not have to become a vegetarian to practice Yoga, but if you wish to practice Yogic ethics, you will continue to make personal choices about what you eat. Many students find, after some practice, that they gradually lose their taste for meat and become vegetarian almost without realizing it. You could actually say that they did not give up meat; meat gave them up. This is what happens when Nonviolence begins to take form.

When I was first beginning to practice Yoga, I did not talk a lot about what I was doing, but word would leak out anyway, especially when people at a dinner party or some other event found out that I was a vegetarian. I never tried to convince anyone else to eat the way I did, and I continue that practice to this day. I believe that this would be an invasion of another person's privacy and thus a subtle form of violence, because I would be demanding that the person be like me.

When pressed about my diet, I tried to explain my views about Nonviolence, trying not to intrude on other people's views. When they asked how I could be sure I was getting enough protein, I could honestly reply that I had studied nutrition and had learned how to count protein grams and adjust my diet accordingly (something I urge anyone to do who wishes to become vegetarian). Some people would insist on continuing: "Well, I'm almost a vegetarian. I only eat fish and chicken. Do you?" Then I would be forced to explain myself further by saying, "No, I never eat anything that looks back." I tried to explain simply that my diet was my own choice, and that, like every other individual, I have a choice about what I want to eat.

I eventually realized that I was unique in that respect. Very few people have a choice about what they eat. Most people eat what is put in front of them, the implication being that they are lucky to have it. Especially during the traditional family holidays, people are expected to eat the traditional fare, not a menu that is chosen for individual taste—not to mention a menu such as mine, which was so often portrayed as exotic then but is becoming so much more common today. My idea is that people get together at holidays to be together, not to eat the same things.

The reasons for a vegetarian diet are much deeper than the simple principle of not causing harm to a living thing. Shaivism teaches that hatred springs from meat and that violence hunts you like an animal, through meat. It goes on to say that the way an animal dies has an effect on you, even if you yourself have not done the actual killing.

Some of the old books on Kashmir Shaivism actually outline three specific crimes against living things (animals or human beings). The first is taking away life, even though the animal or person is innocent and has done nothing to deserve death. The second is the crime of inflicting great pain while killing. And the third is the crime of taking away its strength by trussing it up and tying it down. These old books further say that one has to pay dearly for acts such as these and that it takes 20 lifetimes to pay for such violence. All violence is a result of the spiritual body being ignored, denied expression, and repressed.

I asked Lakshmanjoo once whether these statements are to be taken literally. He said yes, but when I asked if there was anything that one could do to alleviate this penance, he said that according to Shaivite philosophy, the practice of Yoga does help to lessen the burden of repayment. The *Bhagavad Gita* states that anyone who begins serious practice of the ethical guidelines will immediately find relief from the burden of violence in his or her life.

NONVIOLENCE AND LOVE

Love relationships can only approach a real fullness when supported by Nonviolence. I am talking here not only about romantic love but also about the love relationships between parents and children, among friends, and in any other close bond—even a person's love for money, for instance, or work. I do not differentiate among these types of love, because, as I will explain below, love is love.

Most important, love yourself, because this is where violence usually erupts first. It is very clear: If you love yourself, you do not want to harm yourself. Many of our self-destructive behaviors make it look as if we don't love ourselves. When we drink too much, for instance, we are obviously hurting, rather than helping, ourselves.

According to Yoga, love is expressed in the physical body, but love itself is a universal force that belongs to and resides in the spiritual body. It exists unattached to any human relationships.

Love cannot be owned—it can only be used and experienced. As I mentioned above, it is often used self-destructively. You may "love" martinis so much that you want to drink them all day long, but to do so would be using the power of love for self-destruction. Your love for martinis could destroy you. The correct use of love results not in self-destruction, illness, and pain, but in happiness, contentment, and joy. Training in the ethic of Nonviolence will teach you to use love as a tool, checking two things before you act: "Does it hurt me?" and "Does it hurt you?"

Love is so important to us, yet we often bury love's expression beneath our demands and anxieties, such as when we demand that our partners spend more time with us or feel anxious when our children do not call us regularly. This is where the practice of Nonviolence becomes important. Many times we have an image in our minds of what our love relationship should be like. When it does not work out that way, we often blame the other person in the relationship instead of seeing that it is usually our own demands that cause the problem. Demand is considered violent according to Yoga. Naturally, demands cause great unhappiness on both sides.

Whenever you demand that someone conform to your idea of how love behaves, you are causing harm both to that person and to yourself. If you are truly practicing Nonviolence, you would never expect the person you love to be responsible for your happiness. You would realize that love expresses itself in that person in a unique way. If that way is not compatible with your way, it may be an unfortunate situation, but it is not the other person's fault. In fact, I have learned to derive great pleasure from observing the beauty of others' diversity, even if I do not particularly appreciate some of their behaviors.

Consider the love of a child. In most cases, as soon as a child is born, the parents start making demands in the name of love. They want the child to respond, to talk and walk "on time," to be obedient, and so on. We have great expectations for what our children should do and become. How many parents of child prodigies in sports, for example, have been quoted saying something like, "I've been grooming her for this since the day she was born"? In Yoga, this kind of single-minded determination that the child fulfill the parents' wishes would be considered violent because it is very possible that they are not allowing their child to develop into his or her own individuality. We have very little knowledge of what children will do and what they want to become. The gulf between these two perspectives causes great problems.

Real love allows loved ones to be what they are—not the way you think that they ought to be. The tragedy of romance is that most of the time, love is there "if you are the way I want you to be." This is why it is so easy to love pets: They are dependent on us for everything and so their behavior centers around pleasing us—not in becoming what they wish to be. In Yoga, these situations describe a false use of the power of love, not love itself. Even our approach to prayer is usually a barter plan: "If you give me this, I'll give you that"—for example, "If you get me this job, I'll believe that you exist," or "If you let me win the lottery, I'll go to church every week for the rest of my life."

To approach love across a bargaining table would be considered violent, using the power of love for destruction rather than for happiness: "If you do this, act this way, or say these things, I'll love you. If you don't, I won't." Consider the song with the lyrics "When I fall in love, it will be forever, or I'll never fall in love.... And the moment I see that you feel that way, too, that's when I'll fall in love with you." Song after song in our popular music culture extols conditional love as a virtue. To Yogic eyes, this is not love at all, but violence.

Once, in a class about love, I used the film *Wuthering Heights* to point out that the character of Heathcliff didn't actually love the character of Cathy at all. He destroyed her and everything around her with his unrelenting demands and his drive for revenge. Yet I noticed that the first reaction of my class was that this film portrayed one of the great love stories of all time. In the practice of Nonviolence, your whole appreciation of what love is changes to something nondestructive.

Yoga considers all of us to have sprung from the same spiritual source; therefore, by causing harm to another person, we cause harm to ourselves. In any happy relationship, you would never ask someone to do something you are not willing to do yourself. In other words, you would not use the person you love.

The violence in demanding love from another person also has to do with the idea of loving yourself. If I demand that you love me, it means that I am not feeling enough love from myself, and therefore I want you to supply me with what I am lacking. But if I take that quality away from you, who will supply you? In a healthy love relationship, both parties know that they depend on their spiritual selves to supply love for themselves. The supply from the spiritual body is endless; it is freely offered to you for your use, and you can enjoy sharing this.

In a nonviolent love relationship, you bring your own reserves of happiness and strength to the relationship, meeting your lover halfway to complete the union. You are not, then, a dependent, but a strong equal. The relationship is not based on receiving a response from the other person or anyone else but

THE SUBTLE NATURE
OF NONVIOLENCE

Asking someone to do something that you would not do yourself is a subtle form of violence to you and to the other person. Lakshmanjoo was sensitive to this subtle form of violence throughout his life. He told me once that as a young man, he became very upset when his mother served him the best portions of food and gave his guests the less-desirable parts.

LAKSHMANJOO: When there are some guests in front of me, I want to give them good things from my dish and keep second-best things for myself. This is my nature. You cannot change this nature.

ALICE: It gives you happiness, doesn't it?

LAKSHMANJOO: The distributor from the kitchen comes and he keeps good things in my dish and things not so good in dish for others. I hate that. I want to die. Once my mother did this mischief. I was seated in a collection of my spiritual friends, who came to dine with me, and my mother gave me the cauliflower tops. The roots were in their cups. I was so scared, I thought, "I want to die. I don't want to eat that dish." And then I threw that cup and washed my hands and went to my room.

ALICE: Was your mother very upset?

LAKSHMANJOO: She was very upset. I told her, "What are you doing? This is not what I like. I want to serve them first. I would be happy with that." This is my nature, from my very childhood. When I see my friends, I see my spiritual body, and I would never give it leftovers. Love flourishes in this way [quotes from *Bhagavad Gita*]: "Whoever sees my presence in each and every being and who doesn't see my presence only in his personal being; that one who realizes my presence in each and every being, he is residing actually in me [God consciousness]."

simply on the feeling of love springing from your heart. This love exists in full power in your spiritual body and needs no response of any kind; it is self-sufficient. It was here long before you were born, and it will be here long after you are gone. It can never be taken away from you, because you never owned it. According to Yoga, love is universal and not limited by any physical structure or being.

THE POWER TO MAKE A CHOICE

In the previous section, the concept of "not harming yourself" was gradually broadened to include "not harming others" as well, remembering the Yogic principle that everyone springs from the same divine source. As we go on, you will see that both constructive and destructive actions can be transformed by your powers of observation into usable tools for growth. The practice of the ethic of Nonviolence helps you develop your observation skills. As you learn to observe how you harm yourself and others with food, love, and any other situation in life, you will gain the power to make a choice.

Most of us tend to react to situations almost automatically, and so we often do not realize that an action is destructive until it is too late. Automatic reactions have a lot to do with how we were reared. For instance, if your parents told you repeatedly that dogs bite, you may have grown up to hate and fear dogs, even when you learned, as an adult, that most dogs can be quite friendly. Such preprogramming stops the wonderful, spontaneous experiences that the spiritual body can provide. One of the things you learn by practicing nonviolence is how to stop these programmed responses so that each situation becomes new and you can now make a choice as to how to respond to it.

As you become more proficient in your observations, you will be able to apply these concepts to any situation. Because of such constant examination of what you are doing and how you are feeling, your physical body will begin to welcome and trust the emotional contributions of the spiritual body.

The heart, the center of the spiritual body, is where violent qualities such as selfishness and revenge can be transformed. The increased powers of observation that come from practicing ethics clear the path to the heart by teaching you to recognize both the beautiful, powerful use of constructive emotional behavior, which springs from the spiritual body, and the violent result of destructive emotional behavior, which comes from the physical body's reaction when it misconstrues where this emotion comes from. Both are clearly observable when you are trained in ethics. You have a choice. You are no longer helplessly blown about by the winds of indecision. Training in the ethic of Nonviolence helps you make the choice to be constructive or destructive and accept the responsibility for your actions.

Instead of feeling trapped or victimized, you can become very strong as you realize freedom from automatic reactions. You are able to make a new assessment for each situation—is this destructive or is it constructive?—and take the responsibility for your decisions.

This constant observation does not mean that you will develop a passive relationship with the world. On the contrary, Kashmir Shaivism says that this is the only way to be truly dynamic. Practice of the ethic of Nonviolence puts you in the extremely strong mental position of being able to choose what you want to do, because you have carefully examined how this decision will affect you. Most of us want to encourage happy, comfortable, powerful feelings, and through constant examination of what you are doing and how you are feeling, the physical nature gains confidence and welcomes the true emotions of the spiritual body, free of past programming.

Shaivism believes that in order to be really powerful, you have to know yourself, and this means relying on ethical behavior while you decide what it is you really want to say and do in your life. This kind of thoughtful practice protects you from making a great many mistakes and can protect you from a lot of unhappiness.

PROTECTING YOURSELF

When trying to figure out how to choose actions that are not destructive to themselves or others, many people become confused when they encounter situations where they need to protect themselves from harm. Perhaps you, too, are wondering what to do in a situation where you are being threatened.

The standard hypothetical challenge goes something like this: Suppose that you are alone in your house at night and an intruder breaks in and threatens you with a knife. If a weapon were available to you in that situation, would you be justified in harming the intruder in order to protect your own life?

According to Yoga, the simple answer would be that you must do what you have to do in order to protect yourself from harm. A traditional religious idea is that you would die rather than harm another person. In contrast, Yoga would say that your life is as important as anyone else's. Whether or not you have to actually kill the intruder is another story. But this argument only scratches the surface of the reason to practice Nonviolence.

The texts of Yoga go so far as to say that for someone who really practices this ethic of Nonviolence, the power of this ethic manifests itself in a way that might prevent the intruder from showing up in the first place.

The ancient Yogic texts specifically outline the power that is conferred upon the practitioner when that person is established in each ethic. To be "established" in an ethic means that your practice of it is perfect. In the case of Nonviolence, to be established means that you would be incapable of doing anything that would harm yourself or another. In addition, the classic result of becoming established in Nonviolence, as stated in Patanjali's *Yoga Sutras* (see chapter 2), is that then no harm will ever come to you. Nonviolence itself becomes your protection.

Those who practice Nonviolence create an atmosphere of peace around them. Lakshmanjoo translates the verse pertaining to this in one of his books: "No power on Earth can make two mutual enemies enter into combat in the presence of him who,

THE ATMOSPHERE
OF NONVIOLENCE

One moonlit night quite a number of years ago, a friend and I went out into the backyard of my home and sat on the stump of a very large tree that had been cut down—it was at least three to four feet in diameter. Soon a band of little skunks came crawling around the base of the stump, followed by several big raccoons. They all rolled around together. When a large cat arrived on the scene, I expected the cat to chase away all of these little wild animals, or at least cause a fuss. Having three skunks and a cat under your feet could cause real problems! But they all just played around our feet for quite a while as we talked. We were all happy with each other's company. Although we were all different, there was no upset in being together.

being established in subtle Nonviolence, does not harm anyone."

The ubiquitous religious picture that shows the lion and the lamb lying together peacefully implies that there is no hostility in the atmosphere around them and that neither is feeling any hostility or fear toward the other. According to Yoga, those who are successful in Nonviolence create this nonhostile atmosphere wherever they go, and so anyone or anything that enters into their presence is affected by that atmosphere. In reference to our earlier example of the hypothetical intruder, that hostile attitude would be difficult to maintain when confronted by someone who is established in Nonviolence.

Nonviolence creates an ability in you to recognize the underlying unity of life. You then can gain great comfort in realizing that you are not separate or alone, but instead, part of the magnificent system of the world's life. You do not, then, feel threatened by any life form, because any life form would be observed as part of yourself. All life would be your life, supported by the spiritual body.

If you really believe that this is so, you will never fear any situation. Rama told me that one day, when he was living in Kashmir, he was seated on the side of the mountain in meditation when suddenly, he sensed movement to one side. He looked up to see a huge tiger, obviously hungry, creeping past him down the hill. Rama watched as the tiger walked down to a farmer's field, killed a young cow, and dragged it back up the hill, right past where Rama was sitting. It was not unheard of for tigers in those mountains to kill human beings for food, and Rama would certainly have been an easy target—he was alone and unarmed. He believed that his practice of Nonviolence prevented the tiger from attacking him.

DOES A NONVIOLENT PERSON EVER GET ANGRY?

A common misconception about Yoga practitioners is that they are always calm and unruffled, that they never feel or express anger (or any strong emotion). The great Yogis that I have been lucky enough to know would really laugh to even think that they would be described in this way. They were able to express emotion in a pure, very powerful way.

You cannot be human without feeling. Those who pretend that they are not emotional are clearly showing denial of feeling—a complete negation of the power of the spiritual body and its support. Denying feelings is a form of violence against yourself because that egotistical stifling of emotion cannot help but become uncomfortable and cause problems.

Lakshmanjoo made a distinction between anger that was "on the lips" and anger that was "in the heart." A master of Yoga may show anger for a purpose, but the effect is different: The anger will not destroy the recipient. Anger becomes constructive when it is viewed as a friend who reminds you when it is time to protect yourself. It can be a cautionary instrument that serves you.

In most societies, people are taught to subdue and repress anger, along with other so-called undesirable emotions. Someone who practices Yogic ethics believes that all emotions are part of the spiritual body, that they are beautiful and powerful in their own right. They want to show themselves, and you want to welcome them to do it.

I've seen many examples of people who use so-called righteous anger as an excuse for revenge, such as the familiar Hatfield/McCoy feud: "You killed my brother, so I'm going to kill yours." According to Yoga, you harm both yourself and the other person when you do this. Using anger as a weapon to strike out against someone contradicts the idea that anger is a friend who is there to remind you to protect yourself. Thinking or acting on a desire for revenge shows the intrusion of the false ego. This means that you think that you own anger and can force it to do what you want instead of letting it take its own course. Yoga says that the universe has its own way of dealing with injustice. By trying to take on that responsibility yourself, you simply make yourself more uncomfortable and open to pain. As the saying goes, "The mills of the Gods grind slowly, but they grind exceeding fine."

If someone has done something awful to you, you can be sure that it will be taken care of, but you must step aside and let that process function without your interference. It takes experience to practice this, but I can tell you that it removes a great deal of stress to believe that you do not have to take responsibility for the rights and wrongs of the world.

CHAPTER 5

ETHIC #2
TRUTHFULNESS

Don't Lie to Yourself

You probably are aware when you're telling a lie, but can you recognize truth when you hear it? Most of us find it easy to make promises, but we are often lax about following through. Are you able to keep your word, no matter how trivial your promise?

If I were to ask you to describe yourself, you would most likely make many statements that are based on what has been told to you by others. Do you know how to tell what is true about yourself?

The results of practicing the ethic of Truthfulness (in Sanskrit, *Satya*) will begin to show immediately. As you become more aware of the importance of keeping your word, you will experience a growing pride in yourself. You will notice a greater stability in your relationships as your friends learn that they can depend on you. As you learn to recognize what is true about yourself, you will gain great confidence in your abilities and an appreciation for your strengths.

The ethic of Truthfulness has many levels. First, I

> The heart should have
> fed upon the truth,
> as insects on a leaf, till
> it be tinged with the
> color and show its
> food in every...
> minutest fiber.
> (Samuel Taylor
> Coleridge)

will show you how to begin to recognize Truth and how to stop accepting lies about yourself that may contribute to self-destructive behavior. I have designed a fantasy technique that can help you instantly know whether or not a statement about yourself is true. In addition, I will discuss how Truth relates to Nonviolence and the role of differing perceptions in Truth.

Truth is more subtle and hidden than some of the other ethics. For instance, you know right away when you have stolen something, but it is more difficult to recognize Truth. Everyone tries to interpret Truth in his or her own way, and so Truth appears to change in different circumstances when actually it remains the same. As a mundane example, consider the claims made on television for new products, such as household cleansers. The promoter may tell you that this product will clean everything in your house, but you won't know whether or not that is really true unless you try it yourself. This type of consistent observation is necessary to find truth in all things.

THE PROBLEM OF LYING TO YOURSELF

When I first started to teach on the subject of Truth, I asked students to send me examples of lies that had caused problems in their lives. We enjoyed some hilarious examples. One woman wrote about how, as a teenager, she had developed a mad crush on a boy whose only love appeared to be cars. Pretending to enjoy the same interest, she memorized a small amount of information about engines and caught his interest immediately. Love seemed in the offing, but everything fell

A LIE BECOMES "TRUTH"

Sometimes lies seem to become the truth. A student told this story about his experience with truth and lying.

When I was in college, I decided to try telling a big lie in order to watch the results. The opportunity came quickly. I had just traded my car for another one, so I decided that I would tell my college roommate that my previous car had been stolen.

My roommate was skeptical at first, but I had enlisted the help of a close friend to back up my lie, and because two people told it, the lie then seemed more plausible. Eventually, my big lie became a total success. After several days, I noticed a surprising result of this experiment. I found that I was having a difficult time separating the lie from reality. I myself was beginning to believe it. It really frightened me how quickly I lost sight of the truth. Equally frightening is that years later, I sometimes wondered what had happened to my car and the thief who had stolen it.

apart when he invited her to work on his car with him and she had to confess that she knew nothing about cars at all. She never heard from him again.

Another student sent me a newspaper clipping relating an apocryphal story that, some say, has circulated for years. The story concerns a woman who one day looked out of her kitchen window and saw, to her horror, her dog holding a dead rabbit in its mouth. The rabbit looked exactly like her neighbor's pet rabbit. The woman ran outside and succeeded in separating the rabbit from her dog, took it inside, washed it off, and even used her hair dryer to fluff up its fur. After ascertaining that her neighbor was not home, she then put the rabbit carefully back into the neighbor's cage, hoping that the poor woman would think that the animal had died from natural causes.

When the neighbor returned home, she screamed and ran tearfully next door to her friend, crying that her rabbit, which had died that morning and which she had carefully buried in her backyard, had mysteriously come back to haunt her and was lying in its cage in perfect condition.

I relate these stories to get you to think about your own experience with truth and lying and how these experiences make you feel about yourself. How many of you are basing your entire self-image—such as your looks, abilities, accomplishments, and self-worth—on lies told to you by others or by yourself? The self-hate, discontent, and loneliness that I see in so many people is often caused by acceptance of lies told to them by themselves and others.

If you accept lies as true, negative attitudes will grow on your heart like mold. Many debilitating feelings such as fear, insecurity, and anxiety are based on lies—lies that you tell yourself and that you accept from others as true, never having learned how to find out if they are really true. This pattern begins early in childhood. A child doesn't know how to tell what is true and what is not. And so children simply accept what others tell them; they begin to accept lies without question. Eventually, those lies seem to become the truth.

Many people continue accepting lies into adulthood, developing an entire secret inner life that no one ever knows about because it is contrary to what they have been told as children. Thurber's famous story "The Secret Life of Walter Mitty" is a good example. Mitty was raised to live a certain kind of life, which he hated, but he had a completely different, much more exciting life in fantasy. His tragedy was that he could not bring his fantasy into form. He was stuck in the life that he had developed during childhood, a life that did not allow him to portray his true feelings.

External life becomes a superb acting job for people such as Walter Mitty, as they try to become someone they are not in order to fulfill the picture of themselves that a lifetime of lies has created. Meanwhile, their true nature remains hidden. So many people suffer tremendous loneliness because of this pattern. In hiding, they become separate from their real selves, their spiritual bodies.

> He who permits himself to tell a lie once finds it much easier to do it a second and third time, till at length it becomes habitual; he tells lies without attending to it, and truths without the worlds believing him. This falsehood of the tongue leads to that of the heart, and in time, depraves all its good dispositions.
> (Thomas Jefferson)

If people told you, as a child, that you were bad, stupid, ugly, or incompetent, does that make it true? When you place labels on yourself based on lies, you are caught identifying with the physical body and judging yourself according to another person's opinions.

To correctly practice the Yogic ethic of Truth, you must learn to recognize truth in yourself. *What am I doing? What am I saying? What am I seeing? Do I want to be here? Am I saying what I really feel?* Finding the truthful answers to these types of questions, and then acting on them, requires courage. Try to remain aware of your inner conversation constantly. Then use the fantasy exercise described in the next section to test whether or not your statements to yourself are true. As you become proficient in this technique, you will find yourself gaining in strength and confidence because you are building a picture of yourself based upon Truth rather than lies.

HOW TO BEGIN PRACTICING TRUTHFULNESS

Keep your word to yourself and others. This will strengthen your willpower and make you proud of yourself. It will also help you build a reputation of honor in your relationships. If you give your word, no matter how insignificant the issue may be, keep it. Make sure that others can count on your word. Start with small exercises for yourself. If you promise that you will clean the refrigerator this weekend, do it.

Become what you want to be. Do not become a Walter Mitty. Try to make your outer life match your inner fantasy. Refuse to accept lies about yourself, whether told to you by others or by yourself. Appreciate your own strength of being. Try to find out who you really are.

There is an old story that Rama told me about a lion cub whose mother had died and who had been adopted and raised by a flock of sheep. He ate grass, baaed like a sheep, and considered himself a sheep just like the rest of the flock. One night, a lioness crept up and attacked the herd. She killed a sheep and was dragging the body away when she spied the young cub, trembling with fear.

She stopped in her tracks and said, "What are you doing here? You're not a sheep. You're a lion." And she led the cub to a stream where they gazed at their reflections together. The cub saw that he was indeed a lion, not a sheep after all, and he let out a great roar.

Welcome the spontaneity of intuition. Intuition—the spontaneous, creative voice of your spiritual body—cannot speak unless you are listening. Every time you accept a negative statement as true, you are closing the pathway to your spiritual voice. This is because you have allowed your physical body to form a judgment about the truth of the statement on its own. When you invite the spiritual body to speak, you instantly have another option.

Use a fantasy exercise to recognize truth. When I told Lakshmanjoo that I was having difficulty in recognizing what was true about myself, he gave me an answer that always works for me. He explained that Truth can be tasted. It is sweet. I have used this test for many years now with unfailing results.

To try this fantasy exercise, first imagine that the sensation of sweetness is not limited to your mouth but that you can experience sweetness with your other senses as well. Ask yourself how it might feel to experience the sensation of sweetness with something you hear or see. In this fantasy exercise, you will be testing everything you say to yourself by asking if it tastes sweet.

Imagine yourself getting dressed in the morning in front of the mirror. It's not your best day. You look at your reflection and begin to hear yourself talking to yourself in your head. When you become aware of this conversation, give each sentence the test for sweetness: "I look awful"—ask yourself, is this sweet?

"I can't possibly get everything done today"—does this taste sweet?

"If I don't get this project done today, I will certainly be a failure"—and so on.

If the statement does not taste sweet, according to Lakshmanjoo's theory, you can immediately know that it is not true and that this outlook is harmful to you. When thought and behavior are guided by this test for Truth, you can be sure that they will not become self-destructive.

Not all conversation is negative. Once in a while, some of us are lucky enough to look in the mirror and hear, "I look like a million bucks today!" Test this positive thought along with the rest of your inner conversations. Is it sweet? If so, then you know that it is true. As you continue to practice this technique throughout the day, your outlook on yourself will slowly but surely become more positive and constructive because you are telling yourself the Truth.

You can play this fantasy game in your relationships, too. When you are involved in a conversation and someone says something to you that makes you feel uncomfortable, test the statement: Is it sweet? This game will help you avoid pain, because if the person says something to you that causes pain, this test will immediately tell you that it is not true, and so you will be able to protect yourself from harmful reactions.

If you refuse to believe any statement or observation that does not pass the sweet test, you will not be trapped into any position of failure. For instance, a love affair ends, and your former partner tells you that it is all your fault. If you believe this, it will solidify the failure in your own mind. If you use this fantasy sweet test, you will not be trapped. Instead, you have a choice because you know whether or not it is true.

When we think about what is true or not true, we usually try to make decisions with the intellect, which operates from the physical body. Truth cannot be owned by the intellect. The only way the physical body can clearly perceive Truth is by completing a connection with the spiritual body. That connection is encouraged by approaching thoughts and feelings with the fantasy game that I have described above. Move beyond your physical limitation. Test everything with your fantasy exercise by asking, "Does it taste sweet?" If the sweet sensation is not there, do not accept it as true.

THE PERCEPTION OF TRUTH

Most people equate truth with fact. The facts given to us, however, are not always true. For instance, when I was a child, it was considered a fact that the atom could not be split. We now know that this is not true. In addition, the many studies involving eyewitnesses show that even people who supposedly see the same thing perceive it differently. This is because the false ego, which is limited by its connection with the physical body, sees only its own interpretation of events colored by past experience and hasty conclusions.

The false ego believes, "Everyone else thinks as I do." But several people agreeing on an idea does not necessarily make that idea true. There is a famous psychological test in which ten people are put into a room and asked to identify something in the room—let's say, the color green painted on the wall. Nine of the people are secretly instructed to identify the color as blue; the only person who is being tested is the tenth, who usually begins to doubt his own perception and agrees with the other nine people. The subject of the experiment is the will-

JEWELS AND TRUTH

Jewels have been worshiped throughout the ages for beauty and legendary powers. For instance, when emeralds were placed under the tongue, they supposedly forced the person to tell the truth. It was said that celibates can use an emerald to become invisible if they know the trick. Supposedly, sorcerers' magic becomes ineffective when emeralds are worn for protection.

Rubies are said to glow and shine through clothing. Legend says that if rubies are thrown into cold water by the right person, the water will come to a boil immediately. I have never seen this done.

In legend, the sapphire is the jewel that is most closely associated with Truth. If you wear sapphires, eat sapphire dust, or use sapphires in worship, all obstacles between you and Truth are supposedly removed.

When I practiced my discipline of silence in the jungle with Rama, he used to grind up emeralds, pearls, and other gems and feed them to me with deer musk.

ingness to accept a lie as the truth.

If that tenth person practices the Truth ethic, that person probably will not change his or her perception even if it feels embarrassing to stand firm. There is no need to explain or try to convince anyone that one answer is right and another is wrong, because he is relying on the support of his spiritual body, not on outside approval, to tell him what is true. There is no need to proselytize. The proof is for himself alone.

THE POWER OF TRUTH

I have discussed how the acceptance of lies in our past can harm us in the present. Now consider what happens when you

THE POWER OF LANGUAGE

The power of language is illustrated clearly in the wide prevalence of rumors. Many people seem to believe that if a so-called fact appears in print or on the Internet, then it must be true. Indeed, the proliferation of untruth has a frightening commercial quality: It makes money and so it becomes self-perpetuating. Information that is taken as true when it is not is often harmful to the people involved. One example of this is the extensive sensationalistic news coverage of the man suspected—and later cleared—of the bombing in Atlanta during the Olympic games in 1996. His reputation and way of life were irreparably damaged by it.

extend the practice of Truthfulness to your relationships with others. When you begin to recognize truth, it is important to be careful not to use this powerful force to cause harm. Remember to apply all ten of the ethical principles to all your actions. This will help to prevent behavior that is self-destructive or that will cause violence to others.

Many people feel that it is their duty to tell the truth even if it causes pain. Truth then becomes a weapon. The ethic of Nonviolence can be applied to help you avoid causing injury. If you appeal to both your physical and your spiritual bodies before you speak, you can be sure that your expression of truth will be nonviolent. Your physical body makes a judgment based on false ego. Intuition speaks for the spiritual body.

Here is a simple example: You come across an acquaintance you have not seen in many years. Your physical body looks at him and notices that he has gained a lot of weight. Your physical body's false ego says, "It is my responsibility to solve this problem and help this man by telling him my secret to losing weight fast." If you wait for your spiritual body to speak, however, intuition may tell you that commenting on the man's weight would be a violent and unnecessary act.

By appealing to both bodies, you can create a clear channel between the physical and spiritual so that the spiritual body can help you speak without violence. Try this fantasy technique: Imagine a tunnel connecting your physical and spiritual bodies. Try to imagine what happens when that tunnel is blocked. I think that you will realize that neither body can perform competently because half of its power source is cut off. If you can visualize this, you will become aware that this blockage causes pain to both bodies. When you open the channel, you will experience immediate relief.

The story of Cassandra illustrates how truth can be destructive if it is blocked. As a child in the great city of Troy, Cassandra slept in the temple of Apollo, the sun god. Every morning, she was found wound about with snakes, which, by licking her ears, gave her the gift of prophecy and the understanding of the languages of animals.

THE POWER OF TRUTH

Many people would agree that a little truth goes a long way. How many times have you heard people say, "I didn't want to tell the whole truth because it would have been too much for them"? The classical outlook is that truth, in its purest form, is so powerful that it could injure people. Stories such as "The Rose-Colored Glasses" (see page 184) illustrate this point.

Lakshmanjoo told me that when the great sage Patanjali was teaching and lecturing on Yoga, he would sit behind a copper screen to shield his audience from the power of his teaching. It is said that while he was speaking, Patanjali would actually take the form of Kundalini, the spinal nervous system of the spiritual body that is represented by a serpent. And it is believed that without protection, seeing that powerful form would burn the listener to ashes, as if one were standing in the way of a lightning bolt.

THE FORCE OF TRUTH

One of the great depictions of the effect of truth's force is in the film *Satyricon*, in the scene where a hermaphrodite child lies in a dark, quiet cave, resting in a cradle where the special attendants who guard it constantly pour water over the child to keep it comfortable. (The hermaphrodite, half man and half woman, represents the state of God consciousness, or the Universal Body. The child in this story represents the not-yet-fully-developed state of this spiritual force.)

In this scene, two thieves discover the child and realize that it is the source of great power, and so they steal it. They drag it out of the cave and into the sunlight, where, without the protection of the water, silence, and constant nurturing, the brilliant, hot sunlight kills the child. The sun in this story represents the full light of Truth, which the child cannot stand because it is not yet fully developed.

When Cassandra grew to young womanhood, Apollo became so thrilled with her beauty that he took form and tried to make love to her. Because she had been trained as a celibate priestess, she fought him off. Enraged, and unable to revoke her gift of prophecy, Apollo cursed her by causing her prophecies to go unheard. It was Cassandra who recognized the Greeks' wooden horse for what it was, but no one believed her. Cassandra was a channel for truth. When truth was not able to function, its path was blocked, and this caused catastrophe.

TRUTH CAN TAKE FORM

An important aspect of the Truth ethic is to practice being careful about what you say. According to Yogic texts, when you are established in Truth, your words have the power to take shape. It's difficult to maintain this type of constant attention in casual speech. Lakshmanjoo and I discussed this.

LAKSHMANJOO: The result of the discipline of *Satya* [Truthfulness] is that whatever you say comes true. I saw that many times. Whatever you speak, even if you speak just casually, it comes true. It is the power of observing Truthfulness. When the master is the embodiment of Truth, and he tells his disciple, "Oh, you'll be all right; you will realize God," it comes true.

ALICE: The truth itself is so powerful that it takes form, doesn't it? You couldn't impulsively say to someone, "Go to hell." That would be irresponsible, wouldn't it?

LAKSHMANJOO: That is not truth. It is violent truth. It is attack.

ALICE: If you say something like that, would it disturb your own basis of truth?

LAKSHMANJOO: Yes, that is quite true. Also, if you insult truth by joking, that way, you are not in a real sense observing the ethic of Truth.

The extensive use of euphemisms in our language reflects an unconscious awareness that naming a thing will call it into being. In some religions, the name of God is never written or spoken because when that name is uttered, God will take form, and the physical body cannot endure the sight without protection. In the same way, any word that can bring your spiritual body into form must be used with great respect.

TRUTH AND NONVIOLENCE

You have learned how recognizing Truth in yourself can help you avoid self-destructive thought and behavior. We have also discussed how powerful Truth can be, and how easy it might be to use Truth to cause harm unless you remember to consult both your physical and spiritual bodies before you speak. Lakshmanjoo elaborated on the connection between Truthfulness and Nonviolence in our conversation.

LAKSHMANJOO: Truth is that truth which will never hurt anybody's feelings. That is the real truth. He is the embodiment of humility. As Gandhiji said, "The world crushes the dust under its feet, but the speaker of truth should be humbler than the dust."

ALICE: In the Western world, people say, "How can I ever know God? I'm not good enough." And then they say that's humility.

LAKSHMANJOO: That is not humility. That is ignorance. Humility is there; you have to develop it. You have to invoke that humility. This whole universe is not created by God. This universe is actually the commentary of God. So you cannot say, "I am not fit for attaining truth, attaining nearness of God." You are yourself God. You are already there. You have kept yourself away from that by your own choice. By your own ignorance.

Try to recognize when truth is expressed with violence. Lakshmanjoo said, "Be sure the truth you speak is soothing truth. You should see that in that truth, the violence must not come." He told me a story about a sage who was living in the forest. One day, he saw a fawn running fast down the path and, a little later, a hunter. The hunter approached the Yogi and asked if he had seen a fawn pass by and which way it had gone.

The sage answered, "My eyes have seen, but my eyes cannot speak. My tongue can speak, but my tongue has not seen."

In this way, he avoided telling the truth that the hunter was demanding, which would have caused harm to the fawn. This would have been truth with violence.

ALICE: The Truth depends on the Nonviolence?

LAKSHMANJOO: They cannot go away from each other.

CHAPTER 6

ETHIC #3
NONSTEALING

Don't Steal from Yourself
or Others

W hen I refer to stealing in this chapter, I do not mean the most obvious type of stealing, that of material things, but rather the stealing of more nebulous commodities, such as time, attention, power, and confidence. I will be discussing both how we steal from others and, more important, how we steal from ourselves.

What causes the urge to steal in the first place? People feel the need to steal only when they feel lacking in some way. They feel that they are not complete, and so they take from someone else in order to try to become complete.

Stealing from yourself manifests primarily in lack of concentration. As your thought becomes more and more fractured, you will not be able to reach your goals, so you will never become the person you want to be. You have stolen the strength that will help you reach your goal.

For instance, you decide to go on a diet. Your goal is represented by your fantasy of how you want to look. If you are unable to keep up the self-discipline to stay on the diet plan, you are stealing from yourself—your self-sabotage steals the satisfaction of reaching your goal. Practicing the ethic of Nonstealing (*Asteya* in Sanskrit) helps you remain focused on who you are and what you are doing in your life.

When you practice Nonstealing, you develop the knowledge that you already have everything you need or want within yourself. You recognize that although your physical body may feel lacking at times, if you can turn to your spiritual body for what you need, your needs will always be supplied from within yourself. The only way to obtain this complete feeling in yourself is to connect your physical and spiritual bodies by ethical practice. Once you realize that you can depend on your spiritual body to supply all your needs, there is no further compulsion to steal.

Desire is an important aspect of this discussion about stealing because both desire and stealing reflect a feeling of separateness. When you desire something that you think you do not have, you are feeling separate from that thing, and from that desire springs the urge to steal. If you feel a compulsion to have or do a particular thing, try to stop and say to yourself, "By answering this desire, am I stealing? I don't need to steal. I have everything within myself." This constant questioning can help you through many situations.

HOW TO BEGIN PRACTICING NONSTEALING

Learn from the story of Sisyphus. After causing offense to the gods, Sisyphus was sentenced to continually roll a rock to the top of a hill with tremendous effort, after which the rock would immediately roll back to the bottom and he would have to start all over again. He was cursed in believing that he had to do it. He never stopped to figure out why he thought that he had to do it. His mental conversation told him to do it and he never changed that inner conversation.

How many things do you do because you think that you must do them? This is clearly a case of stealing from yourself by holding on to a belief system that is false. The story of Sisyphus describes a human being whose false ego is operating. Sisyphus says, "I have to roll this rock up the hill." What would happen if he didn't believe this? He would be free from the curse. Similarly, the false ego believes that success means physical fulfillment of an unending stream of desires. You have to do this, you have to have that, or you're never going to make it. This is exactly the curse that Sisyphus carried: "I have to do it." This puts all the responsibility on the physical body.

What if that were not true? When you feel the compulsion to do something, try to observe the false ego operating in your physical body. If you can do this, an alternative from your spiritual body will appear almost immediately. It is similar to consulting a well-respected doctor for a second opinion about a medical condition. By waiting for the spiritual body to speak, you realize that you have another choice.

Put this idea into action the next time you notice yourself saying, "I have to do this." First, quiet yourself. Then ask yourself, "What would happen if I did not do this?" Listen for the voice of your spiritual body, which will offer an alternative.

Practice small deprivations. Try taking something small away from yourself and experiencing a good result from it. For example, give up desserts for a week and perhaps you will notice an improvement in how you look and feel. Or give up that third cup of coffee and maybe you will gain a greater feeling of relaxation.

By taking something inconsequential away from yourself, you will find that it is replaced immediately. In the simple examples above, the replacements were new emotional confidence and the ability to relax. Continuing this type of investigative

INTERNAL ROBBERS

Lakshmanjoo calls unchecked thoughts thieves of the mind, saying that they deprive the practitioner of valuable awareness and concentration by creating a screen of random distractions that break one's awareness.

play will help demonstrate to you that you do not need to steal at any time.

Practicing being in need of some small thing and learning that you do not have to steal to fill that need shows you that your needs are answered from within yourself by your spiritual body. When you take something away from yourself, watch very closely to see what is supplied in its place. As the saying goes, nature abhors a vacuum.

Observe your inner conversation. The ultimate stealing from yourself is unchecked mental conversation. Oftentimes, as you become focused on a thought, something else will arise in your mind to steal your attention. This constant stealing prevents full concentration. A person who has lost concentration has trouble completing any task, and so the fluctuation of concentration can be seen as a type of self-torture, a self-destructive attitude that often goes unnoticed.

Stealing, then, in the ultimate sense, is a common state functioning heartily in yourself against yourself. Take a moment to answer these questions: What am I stealing from myself? What am I allowing my thought patterns to steal from me? What am I stealing from my life by my thoughts?

Practicing the ethic of Nonstealing helps you escape from being blown about by the wind of impulse, mindlessly responding to every whim and compulsion, which can become destructive. You have the strength of conscious choice and the awareness of both the consequences and the rewards of your choices.

THE PRINCIPLE OF DESIRE

Desire is a natural primitive feeling. The world runs on desire: the desire to live, to mate, to eat, and to protect one's territory. Every breath you take is an expression of your desire for life. Yogic literature considers the creative cycles of the entire universe to be based upon the attraction—the mutual desire—between male and female principles of consciousness.

What connects desire to stealing is the physical body's compulsion to fulfill desire at any cost, which means taking from someone else—or yourself. When you are practicing the ethic of Nonstealing, it is important to closely observe your desires and the actions you take to fulfill them. Desire can then become an important tool in reaching your goals.

Desire also has an expansive quality because it promotes change. The physical body uses desire as a whip because the physical body expects itself to answer all desire. But it can't do that, and so it often suffers great stress. When desire is given to the spiritual body, however, no effort is involved, and no stress is produced. The spiritual body supplies the answer to all desires effortlessly. All you have to do is remember where the gift came from.

THE POWER OF DESIRE

The power of attraction shows everywhere around us. Artists and decorators know that certain colors complement other colors. Chemists know that certain substances react harmoniously with other substances. Cooks know that certain spices go best with certain foods. Water automatically finds its level—you could say that it longs for it, looks for it, runs to it. All these are examples of the principle of desire in action.

The connection between desire and stealing can be demonstrated in two important areas of life that I also discussed with regard to the ethic of Nonviolence: food and love.

DESIRE AND FOOD

Eating is a natural, primitive function, and it is always based in desire. We desire food either because our bodies are in need of sustenance or because the food looks and smells very tempting. We usually do not consider where the food comes from or what exactly is responding to our desire.

One of the problems the physical body encounters as it acts to obtain food is that the food must be protected so that no one else will steal it. In common hospitality, food is always offered to visitors. This ancient, primitive custom arose because of the belief that the visitor, having been appeased, will not steal from you.

On the other hand, history also shows that satisfying the guest's desire for food is a way of putting the guest off guard so that the host can take advantage of the person. When satiation of desire is reached, people become vulnerable.

Ethical training advises you to observe food—everything, in fact—as divine gifts from your spiritual body. This attitude eliminates the frantic grasping and guarding of the physical body, because you begin to know that food is supplied by your spiritual body, and so you don't have to worry about getting it, keeping it, preserving it, or protecting it. Your physical body will still perform its food-related functions of shopping, cooking, and eating, but you will realize that you are not alone, that your spiritual body is also involved. By continually recognizing the participation of your spiritual body in this very basic function of eating, you will eat better and be more nourished because you have the strength of two bodies to make wise choices.

DESIRE AND LOVE

Love relationships, like our need for food, are inevitable, a natural fact of life. Yet most relationships are based upon what

A NEW EXPERIENCE OF LOVE

My own experience of love, in the many years since I have been practicing these ethical principles, is much more exciting and far beyond the narrow version of love that is portrayed in magazines and on television. If you'd like to experience this type of love, here is an easy exercise to try: Sit still and quiet. Let your mind fantasize about love and all its possibilities. Then simply stop all thought and observe what happens. This will encourage your spiritual body to show you a different type of love, a love that exists free from any shred of demand.

you can "get" from the other person and what the other person can get from you. This type of relationship implies a demand, which is a form of stealing. Some examples are relationships in which one partner demands constant attention from the other, when one partner is always in the role of comforter or nourisher, or when a partner subtly or overtly demands that the other partner change in some way to conform to a fantasy ideal. The other partner in these examples is a victim of stealing: the stealing of time, attention, identity, or strength. They have simply been used as a vehicle to fulfill a fantasy of desire.

Most of us want to give of ourselves to people we love, and it is hard to refuse a needy partner whom we love, but this type of relationship will not last, because no one can give continually without replenishment.

Love, when based in ethical conduct, makes no demands because each partner's needs and desires are met internally, through the spiritual body. Whatever they may lack is constantly replenished from within. This means that each can be responsible for his or her own happiness. There is no need to demand comfort, praise, attention, or anything else from the other person.

The relationship becomes a true partnership of two people who love each other as they are, without conditions. Both partners contribute support to keep the relationship strong. In other words, the love relationship does not have to depend on one or the other person, because it draws strength from both parties.

If you can approach nondemanding love through the ethic of Nonstealing, you will experience great peace. The absence of desire gives you rest, and the participation of your spiritual body constantly and effortlessly renews your participation in the relationship.

THE RESULT OF NONSTEALING

Yogic texts state that the great power gained by mastering the ethic of Nonstealing is that "all luxury will automatically be at your disposal." In other words, by observing the great force of desire, you can make a conscious choice about your behavior. If you can do this, eventually everything you need or want will automatically be supplied to you by your spiritual body.

This is a very unusual way of thinking for those of us who have been taught that everything we get is supplied by our own efforts—in other words, physical efforts of the physical body. In practicing the ethic of Nonstealing, you can recognize that it is the spiritual body that is the source for all fulfillment of desire.

When you have mastered the ethic of Nonstealing, you do not have to constantly protect your belongings, because it is impossible for anything to be taken away from you. Rama told me about an experience he had while living in a cave above Rishikesh, a hill station high in the Himalayas above Haridwar. One day, he went for food and returned several hours later to find a young man standing stock-still, rooted to the floor inside the cave, his arms filled with Rama's few belongings: a water

CAREFUL CHOICES

Lakshmanjoo told me, "Someone who does not practice the ethic of Nonstealing just gets piled up in junk." What a wonderful way to say that careful choices in life are needed. Many times, what you end up with is not what you wanted at all.

pot, a small carpet, and several books.

Upon seeing Rama, the man cried out, "Oh, Sir, please release me! I came here to steal, but I have been unable to move these past hours!"

Rama calmly assured the young man that he could have whatever he wanted if it would ease his sorrow, and that he, Rama, was not the one holding him there against his will. (The power of Rama's achievement in Nonstealing was actually holding the young man there.) Rama then released the man, who was then able to move. He put down what he had attempted to steal, bowed deeply to Rama, and took his leave.

EVERYTHING IS A DIVINE GIFT

The power of Nonstealing is based in the remembrance that everything comes from God. Lakshmanjoo said, "Always remember the fact that in practicing such a difficult art as ethical behavior, you are approaching God consciousness. The first thought in your mind upon receiving anything would be 'This has come from God. God has sent this to me.' The idea that everything comes from God is a transformation of the laws that surround it."

In other words, everything we have is a divine gift, and we can observe it all with wonder, delight, and astonishment. There is no fear of losing anything. In the same way, if everything is at your disposal, you don't feel the need to steal from anyone. A great feeling of peacefulness surrounds a person who knows this. If you have everything, you are never in need.

SECRECY AND STEALING

Secrecy is an insidious form of stealing that I sometimes see in people who believe that keeping things hidden is equivalent to behaving ethically because they are not causing upset to others. Secretiveness steals time and attention from others because it forces them to spend a long time figuring out what you are really trying to say and who you really are.

I do not encourage secretive behavior. For you great romantics who enjoy secrecy, I suggest that your vocabulary is limited. I think that you can find ways to be romantic and direct. If your thought is more enjoyable in secret, then keep it there. But be careful not to use this attitude in revenge. Anything worth knowing is worth seeing. Ethical behavior teaches you to be direct and truthful about what you say and do.

CHAPTER 7

ETHIC #4
CELIBACY

Be Respectful and Aware of Sexual Desire in Yourself

Many of you are probably planning to skip this chapter because Celibacy is not a popular word in the United States. It is a frightening term to most people, especially those who suffer from a broken heart, because they think that if they practice Celibacy, they will be removed from the sweet support systems of life: touching, love, companionship, the enjoyment of a relationship. They look upon celibacy as a tragic, suffering sacrifice, like living in a convent with bare feet on cold stone floors. This is not at all what the ethic of Celibacy is about. If you can gather up your courage and read on, you may find that the subject is not so daunting after all.

Celibacy (or *Brahmacharya*, in Sanskrit) can be used as a building block to make you wonderfully free, to give you time to observe yourself and withdraw to your inner self, enabling you to rest and renew and then come forward again in full strength. In the practice of Celibacy, you can learn how to enjoy the feeling of sexuality without the constant fear that you will lose it—or the need to depend on anyone else to provide it.

HOW TO BEGIN PRACTICING CELIBACY

Start with five minutes a day. Celibacy can be practiced for very small periods at first. I am not talking about years of abstinence. If you would like to try this practice, you may choose any length of time that you prefer, but my suggestion is that you start with a very short period: perhaps five minutes a day.

Plan a time for this five-minute experiment when you are by yourself. The type of celibacy that I am talking about here is restraint of the sexual conversation of the mind. During your five minutes of celibacy, the idea is not to indulge in mental fantasy about sex.

This type of celibacy can be practiced by anyone, and no one needs to know that you are doing it. If you are currently involved in a sexual relationship (with someone other than yourself), there is no need to hurt your partner by violently announcing that you are withdrawing yourself from sexual involvement.

If you restrain your thoughts for five minutes and intently observe them, you can clearly see how pervasive sexual thought is in your mental pattern. This brings on an intense awareness of your inner thinking mechanisms. It becomes a very simple task to notice sexual conversation in your mind. Once you start practicing this small exercise, you can then realize that all your actions, day and night, are subject to this sexual content, and that your behavior is being affected accordingly.

In order to practice the Celibacy experiment correctly, you must set a definite starting and ending time, whether five minutes, one day, or whatever time period you choose, and see if you can complete it. Try not to set a goal that will be too hard to reach.

A RESTFUL NEW OUTLOOK

I used to give a lecture on my book *The Joy of Celibacy*. I'll never forget the time when I gave this talk to employees of a heavy-equipment manufacturing company in southern Ohio and afterward overheard one of the participants leaving the auditorium saying, "Geez, can you imagine how restful that would be—five minutes not thinking about broads!"

There is a great difference, however, between involvement and ownership in sexual thought. If you are practicing Celibacy, you pull back from involvement with sexual thought. This does not mean that you do not have any thoughts about sex; it means that you watch thought operating without becoming involved. You will find that you can watch other people involved in sexual play and conversation with a great deal of enjoyment.

Go out on Friday night, and just watch. Enjoy sexuality expressing itself. Observe its power. Listen to what it says. Try to understand how people feel, but only in a very private way, in your own observations.

In this way, you will begin to appreciate the fact that sexuality expresses itself in everything. The basis of sexual power is represented in the deity of Earth Mother herself, the manifestation of all creation. It is the power that keeps you alive. You cannot get away from it. As the philosophy of Kashmir Shaivism says, you do not try to run from it, you try to join with it.

If you were able to sustain this expansive idea about sex, sexual experience would give you an awareness of its magnificence in such a way that sexual behavior would no longer be commonplace. Your awareness of the connection of the ecstacy of sex with this magnificent quality that is the essence of life itself, and the universal force that underlies it, brings a new dimension to all sexual relationships. There is no more fear of

THE POWER OF CELIBACY

It is said that the great god and hero Krishna was a practicing celibate and yet he had 1,800 wives. On top of that, he would make love with anyone he met. Both men and women were entranced by him. The most notable quality of Krishna was that he never worried about being able to satisfy so many people. He was always sure of his potency. I think that those who have practiced periods of Celibacy for quite a long time become very sure of themselves, not only in sexual performance but in all performance.

How could Krishna practice Celibacy perfectly while simultaneously making love with so many people? Krishna's physical body was extremely active, but he was functioning completely from his spiritual body, so there was never any loss or harm in what he did.

There is a story about someone who once challenged Krishna's performance of Celibacy. This man and Krishna were waiting to cross the great river Jumna, which was swollen with floodwaters and very deep and treacherous. Krishna called on the river to verify his perfect practice of Celibacy. He said, "If Krishna has practiced Celibacy perfectly, may the river part and become a road." Thereupon the waters of the river immediately drew back on either side and became a dry road for them to cross. (This story may remind you of the Old Testament story of Moses parting the Red Sea. Is it possible that Moses was teaching the same discipline? We do not know, but we do know, according to Shaivism, that intellectual understanding of Celibacy is impossible; it must be experienced.)

loss, and no more loneliness. You do not have to have a sexual partner to recognize that the basic power of sexuality lies within you; it is not dependent upon any other person.

Expand your practice time. Once you become comfortable

with the five-minutes-a-day commitment to Celibacy, increase your practice to perhaps one day a month or one day a week. Now you begin to watch not only your mind but also your body. Many people have the mistaken idea that simply because they have not knowingly indulged in sex during that time, they have been celibate. The practice of Celibacy must have a precise be-

EXPERIENCES WITH CELIBACY

One morning, a student of mine decided that he wanted to try a period of Celibacy. I said, "That's fine. When are you going to start?"

He replied, "I'm going to start today and go for three days."

That evening, when he came to our house for dinner, he asked if he could talk to me. He did not want to talk in front of anybody else, so we went down into the basement. At that time, I was living in a big old rambling house with a maze of dark rooms in the basement.

I can remember him looking at me over the furnace pipes, saying, "I want you to know that I couldn't keep my Celibacy commitment. When I left here this morning, I drove out of the driveway and oddly enough, an old girl-friend, whom I hadn't seen for several years, was standing at the corner waiting for a ride, and it was all over." We both laughed, realizing that this commitment to even three days of celibacy was a bigger task than he had suspected. After five or six attempts, he finally made it through one day.

Then there was the couple who decided to practice Celibacy for a time together and thought that if they engaged only in mutual masturbation, they were fulfilling their promise of celibacy. This is not what we are describing here. Celibacy means that you do not indulge the body in any sexual action.

ginning and ending date. A certain time is set aside for this practice. Then the fun begins!

Most of the students I have known have been unable to keep that commitment for more than a couple of hours in the beginning. You can expect to lose many times before you succeed. It takes practice and it takes a great sense of humor.

Although you will not be personally involved in sex during your commitment to Celibacy, you can still constantly enjoy the observation of it while not owning it. I remember a religious man I once met on an airplane who, when he traveled, had himself blindfolded so he would not lay eyes on a woman. This kind of behavior is not at all connected to Yoga.

THE RESULT OF PRACTICING CELIBACY

Small periods of Celibacy help to build the spiritual body, and the result of this united body, physical and spiritual together, is described by Lakshmanjoo: In his words, Celibacy refers to the maintenance of mental and physical character. "Maintenance" in this context means pulling back from relationships that sacrifice your personal power. Why is it important to cultivate this aspect of one's character? Because it allows you to attain *viryalabha*, the storage of power.

Yogic texts say that the result of practicing Celibacy is that "your word becomes true." Lakshmanjoo elaborated on this by saying that this practice gives you strength for spiritual growth. This means that it will support the spiritual body that you are inviting to emerge.

Lakshmanjoo also said that in the later stages of Celibacy—after you have practiced on and off for quite a while—the awareness that you have a choice in your sexual attitude begins to come to you. He says clearly that this knowledge is not meant to be used in debates or to impress others with a show of understanding but is meant for the pursuit of

God consciousness, which is then easily attained. It is said that if someone who is practicing Celibacy correctly is instructed in meditation by his or her teacher, meditation will bring results easily and quickly. In other words, the practice of Celibacy supplies what you need to bring the spiritual body's form into view.

Lakshmanjoo and I discussed the practice of Celibacy one day in his garden.

> LAKSHMANJOO: *Brahmacharya* [Celibacy] gives power in your body. Your power is maintained.
>
> ALICE: So whatever you say comes true?
>
> LAKSHMANJOO: Yes. When rise of God consciousness takes place, you know what kind of joy [the Yogi] experiences: that utmost joy of God consciousness, which is just like the joy of sexuality.
>
> ALICE: Is that the supreme sexual feeling that you talk about?
>
> LAKSHMANJOO: Yes. And that sexual feeling is never lost. It is not just sexual feeling for two minutes or three minutes only and then it is gone. Not that. It is that sexual feeling that is everlasting. Only you think that you are away from it. It is always there. So maintaining that *Brahmacharya* in yourself gives power to that joy.
>
> ALICE: So then sexual joy is not transitional; it's constant?
>
> LAKSHMANJOO: Yes. If you are given to that outer sexual joy, that inner sexual state begins to become less and less. So [the practice of] *Brahmacharya* is a must. Breath stops and you get internal flow. Then that sexual joy is just like a fountain.

Who says Celibacy is dull? What Lakshmanjoo is describing is the ultimate experience of God consciousness. He told me that if you multiply the ecstatic feeling of a sexual orgasm by a million times, that might approximate the feeling of sexual joy that is experienced in God consciousness. He also said that this ultimate experience cannot be sustained by a human body, so at first it comes on little by little, incrementally. This is why you will never see a true Yogi who looks unhappy. The outlook on sexuality of someone who has had even a taste of this experience changes completely.

A perfect illustration of this experience may be found in the beautiful verses of the *Song of Solomon*. It sounds like a love poem between a human man and woman, but from a mystical point of view, this poem describes the male/female attraction and the complexity of the universe that results from their joining. It is about your joining with yourself, opening the door to the tremendous expression of individuality that pours through you as you meet yourself. This experience has its own music and conversation.

When you have found yourself, you can never lose love. There is no loss because love lies within you, and the love of yourself *for* yourself never leaves. You can never lose it by loving someone else, and you never depend totally on someone else to provide love to you. If celibacy has only one virtue, it is to protect you from loss while you transform that loss with courage. This, then, carries a new expansion of joy and freedom into your relationships. You are not going into a relationship empty-handed, and you are not haunted by the specter of loss. You are bringing something to the relationship, not expecting someone else to be the main contributor. In other words, you can carry the responsibility of your involvement in all phases of a relationship without fear.

HEALING A BROKEN HEART

Celibacy can be used to heal a broken heart. I use the phrase "broken heart" to mean any feeling of loss, separation, or sadness. It is not limited to the pain of a failed love affair or marriage. If you have lost your job, for instance, or someone you love has died, or you are faced with a serious illness, you feel a loss of power and a sense of impotence—symptoms of a broken heart. Often, people equate the feeling of failure with a broken heart, but to me, a broken heart is a much more serious condition.

Frequently, people approach Yoga during times of crisis, when their lives seem to be in such a mess that they are desperate to find something to make it better. It is more difficult, however, to practice Yoga with the distractions a broken heart can bring, because Yoga demands full attention. And if you are suffering from a broken heart, the wound is so painful that you cannot concentrate on anything else except the pain. The practice of Yogic ethics, however, especially small periods of Celibacy (even five to ten minutes a day), helps to heal that wound in you and allows you to bring yourself back into balance so that the experience of Yoga can come on freely and become a support for the future involvements of your life.

I have found that small periods of Celibacy are extremely helpful for people experiencing divorces or any relationship losses. It is very clear to me that during times of extreme stress, people need to protect themselves against loss of energy in relationships. They need to protect their strength and privacy, and very few relationships are set up to do this. Celibacy allows you an inner place to hide and heal.

Many times, people who have suffered a loss try to fill the empty space right away with a new relationship—even if it is potentially self-destructive, such as the Friday-night pickup scene—or surround themselves with material things. This kind of "self-medication" can never last. The casual sexual relationships that so many people enter into, for whatever reason, usually result in a loss instead of a gain. I believe that the feeling of loss can only be replaced by the individual turning inward for strength and protection. The real healing comes from within yourself, and Celibacy protects you while that wound heals. Gradually, you realize that your strength has always been there within you. This realization provides strength for your re-entry into self-satisfying relationships.

Celibacy allows a person to find depth and meaning in relationships of all kinds, from the most intimate sexual relationships to the most impersonal social relationships. The male/ female principles of the universe are always longing and searching for each other. With Celibacy we begin to realize that this whole picture of the universe is encompassed in ourselves, and that the most important relationship is between our two halves: our inner and outer beings—the spiritual and physical bodies.

In Yoga, unlike religious traditions, Celibacy is presented without any moral attachments. It is practiced simply to achieve a particular result: the powerful unity of the individual. Brief periods of Celibacy can vastly increase peripheral awareness, which is an important factor in making meaningful life choices. When you practice Celibacy, you develop increased sensitivity to your new ability to make choices in your sexual relationships. This is because most sexual relationships are based on impulse and, therefore, often become self-destructive. Thus, Celibacy creates truly mature adults who take responsibility for their own happiness.

I like to think of Celibacy as a basic, perfect protection that we can call on in ourselves at any time and that we can return to in rest and observation. It has an atmosphere that is noninvasive and peaceful, a place where we can remember the total protection we experienced in the unborn state—floating, dreaming, all needs provided.

RECOGNIZING LOVE

I have found periods of Celibacy to be extremely useful in finding and recognizing love in my life. Love means everything to me, and I have noticed that love seems to be important to everyone else in this country as well, even in the business world. Americans not only want to do business but they also want to be liked, bringing an added dimension to negotiations that is rarely understood by representatives of other countries.

Celibacy can also improve sexual relationships because the new awareness removes the subliminal fear of loss and impotence so pervasive in today's society. One experiences a beautiful depth in love relationships as one learns to communicate in the hundreds of ways that sexuality provides. In Yoga, sex is viewed as the beautiful, powerful basis of human life. The person who enters into a relationship with some Celibacy training will be more aware of this, and it will add great enjoyment to relationships. How does this happen? When a relationship of great meaning appears, do you have the power to become involved or are you afraid to take the step? Have you wasted your real energy on things that do not matter?

SEX, CELIBACY, RELIGION, AND SOCIETY

Our culture is pervaded by contradictory views of sex and celibacy. Sex is both celebrated as the source of life itself and degraded as evil and sinful. Celibacy is usually associated with religious disciplines and is often presented as the only way to become "pure" enough for spiritual experience. At the same time, it is presented as a hardship and a severe discipline.

Celibacy has been presented by the church as a vow of separation from the strongest force of life: sexuality. It is a vow taken for life, never to be changed—a feat that is, in fact, nearly impossible, because it insults the primitive quality of life itself. In demanding Celibacy, the church implies that the only pure love is love for God, and that love has nothing to do with sex. Consider the "purity paddles" that young seminary students are given to use for tucking in their shirttails so as to avoid touching their genitals with their hands.

The logical conclusion is that loneliness, denial, and suffering are ultimately good for you, and that God wants that product through you because if you live through it, and can stand it long enough, you will become not divine, perhaps, but nearer to God. The church has a perfect right to say what it wishes in constructing its creed, of course. And for some people—a very few, I would guess—it may work. But most of us are much more body-oriented and attuned to our natural instincts.

It is unfortunate that Celibacy has been given such a negative aura in this way. Religion has no ownership of the use of Celibacy, but religion has realized the power that can be obtained from individuals willing to allow this pilfering of personal strength. Celibacy, which could be such a valuable tool for American society, is being ignored, lost to us, secreted away like the Dead Sea Scrolls to be revealed only selectively. Sexuality lies within us, ready to flow and show its hand in all its beauty and even speak its poetry and song, but it is held back by the cork of fear and guilt, cheating society of the full impact of using whole, strong persons to express it.

A common social and religious outlook says that the only way to approach God is through self-denial. This attitude can result in terrible suffering as both men and women feel the pressure to continually give and give, sacrificing their own lives for community or church with no time for family or self-renewal. Basing your entire life on experiences of loss results in a life that soon becomes empty and unfulfilling. I believe that life should be lived with an attitude of replenishment, with time and energy to observe the joy and beauty that lie around us. To become strong and powerful individuals, we must maintain our well-being. We must learn how to repair our losses. Small periods of Celibacy are a way to do this.

Many people believe that celibacy is a type of loss so horrible that they cannot even consider it. One of the many translators of Patanjali's *Yoga Sutras* says in his commentary, "Of all the virtues enjoined in *yama-niyama*, [Celibacy] appears to be the most forbidding, and many earnest students who are deeply interested in Yogic philosophy fight shy of its practical application in their lives because they are afraid that they will have to give up the pleasures of sex indulgence." You can see that the specter of sex is linked to fear, loss, and "giving up."

Fear of loss is rampant in our world. "Use it or lose it" was the watchword of the 1950s and 1960s. So many people that I

GOD IS NOT SEPARATE FROM ANYTHING

In the mid-1960s, while in Yogic training with Rama in the jungle above Haridwar, I often saw people who had retreated to the area to perform harsh penances to "purify" themselves in order to reach God, as if God were separate from them, only appearing in suffering.

Our compound was situated on the bank of the Ganges River, and one day, I watched a man taking his stand in the river to pray, raising his arms to the sun. I was horrified when I saw blood running down his legs into the freezing water. At first, I thought that he had been injured and ran toward him to help. He retreated rapidly, stumbling over the stones in the river, trying to get away from me. I stopped as I realized that he was avoiding me because I was a woman, the very source of sin from which he was trying to escape. He had wrapped brambles around his genitals and legs so that the slightest erection would cause bleeding and pain. I remember Rama laughing and saying, "These people have the wrong idea. God is not separate from anything."

know have had to deal with problems of impotence—men and women alike—all based on fear of loss. Fear of loss can only occur when you think that you own something, an attitude that is a function of the false ego. If you can become aware of who you are and what you are and the power that you have, fear of loss does not imprison you. The spiritual body provides an unlimited supply of what you need.

SEXUALITY IN YOGA

As a Yogi trained in the Shaivite tradition, I am interested in connecting with my innate spiritual nature. I think that this magnificent, primitive treasure of sexuality in ourselves is not only often ignored but, in fact, openly disdained. I firmly believe that a powerful individual is of much more use to religion and society than a suffering dependent.

In Yoga, and especially in the tradition of Kashmir Shaivism, sex and Celibacy are presented in an entirely opposite manner from the societal attitude of shame and aversion. Shaivism considers sexuality and Celibacy as the main source of strength in one's personality. Sexuality can never be denied, and its beautiful qualities are often described incorrectly. There is no judgmental quality of sexuality in Yogic philosophy, only appreciation and awareness of its power. As Yoga students become more and more aware of the force of sexuality, they can begin to realize its constant strength and support.

SOME EXPERIENCES OF STUDENTS

Let me share with you some of my students' experiences with Celibacy. Each one is unique and deserves comment.

Several months ago, I started having a recurrent vision. Just before dropping off to sleep, a giant male hand would reach down and pick me up by the crotch just as if my body were a suitcase. I would have this feeling of being lifted slightly off my bed, hips higher than the rest of my body, and only then would I go to sleep. This would happen several times a week. I began to get the idea that my life was out of control in this area.

About a week before this class, I decided that I could not practice Yoga or pursue anything more until I took care of a rampant desire in me to be with a male counterpart. Then, of course, I found out that your class was on—what else—Celibacy. I became hysterical. I cried. And so did all the friends that I told when they realized the irony of the situation.

I find my life to be relatively worthless without this play between the sexes. Not just physical sex, but the mental and emotional joining and the talking and the fun. Most of all, I have this ideal picture of this perfectly balanced, joined couple in total harmony with one another.

This primitive vision of perfect harmony between male and female is the very picture of the experience of Yoga when the female principle of action joins with the male principle of support. This joining, called the Universal Body or God consciousness, can only exist within you. Whether you are a man or a woman, the perfectly harmonious picture of a love relationship that is facing you is a picture created by your own fantasy.

Fantasy has never been looked upon as an important tool for our lives. In fact, many times, people are scolded because their relationships with their fantasies seem to take them away from the reality of their lives. Ethical behavior can protect you from this type of potentially destructive fantasy.

If fantasy does not take form and remains privately hidden in the mind, it can never be shared. It takes courage to be yourself. Bringing your fantasy into form shows the other person who you really are, not just how you look. In other words, your deepest feelings about love can be easily displayed in your personality. This creates a very different kind of relationship from impulsive physical attractions, which end up with both partners realizing that they don't know the other person at all. Bringing fantasy into form constructively means that you can be your whole self; you can act out your fantasy safely, guided by the ethical practice of small periods of Celibacy.

So, do you need only one relationship? Can you see how you could walk around looking at everyone and being extremely happy sexually? If you make love with someone, fine. And if you don't, fine. That is how Krishna (see "The Power of Celibacy" on page 92) functioned. He had no fear of losing anything because he was perfectly aware that love was there with or without his involvement. This is an entirely different outlook from "someday, my prince will come." In other words, you are not depending upon happiness to be provided to you from outside sources.

Try practicing Celibacy. You will become very sensitive to feelings that, up until now, you may have ignored. And you will realize that those powerful feelings do not depend on anyone else. By becoming more and more connected with your source of feelings, which is your spiritual body, and following this ethical guideline, you will eventually see yourself as extremely powerful—and I doubt that you would have to prove your sexuality or power to anyone.

The idea behind the practice of Celibacy is not to be in need but to enjoy the observation of sexuality so much that physical involvement becomes a secondary issue. This takes subtlety. If you went to a party, you could have a terrific time because you could enjoy the sexuality of everyone there without any physical involvement by yourself or anyone else. You would simply enjoy the beauty and power of it.

> After resuming an active sexual life in a love relationship, I found my appreciation for sex was greater, although my need was relatively decreased. It seems now that I have less of a tendency to lose myself during a sexual encounter. I think that this is a by-product of Celibacy.

Absolutely not! When you are involved in a great love affair, are you thinking about how you feel in that love affair all the time? If you are, you cannot call it a love affair; you should call it an ego affair. In a real love affair, you are thinking about the other person. You have lost all thought of yourself. That is why a love affair is so great. You have lost all thought of what you need and what you're doing in the complete enjoyment of this union. Obviously, this student has an incorrect view, because the practice of Celibacy would allow complete enjoyment in the other person's actions without any loss to yourself. The bottom line appears to be that the love affair that this person is involved in is obviously not satisfying. What do you think about when you're making love?

When my wife was pregnant, several months went by when we didn't have any sex because the doctor advised against it, so it was a sort of "forced" celibacy. I found that waves of sexual desire would hit me and, at first, cause me a lot of grief. One night, I was watching TV when a sexual desire just came over me. It was so overpowering, I could hardly stand it. And then I realized that I really didn't have to do anything about it. For the first time in my life, I just sat there and enjoyed the feeling. And it was the most incredible experience that I've ever had in my whole life.

When the sexual feeling came over this man, he was able to observe it and enjoy it without acting on it. There was no feeling of loss, deprivation, pain, or demand—simply an enjoyable experience.

MY EXPERIENCE WITH CELIBACY

My sex education consisted entirely of my mother saying, "Sex is a big thing." No one talked to me about love, but it bloomed from within me, so I dreamed on. I took it for granted that if I married someone, both love and sex would be mine. I think perhaps that I left home to find love. I was young, only 18, when I married.

I probably would still be moving within the whirlwind of need and loneliness around me, but in my mid-twenties, my husband left me. I was a young mother with two sons. I don't mean that he left me by walking out; he left me by turning his attention to other women. It was the same old American ailment, the double standard of existence: Feel one way, act another. We continued to act as if we were still a couple, going to parties, doing the same things we did before, but how difficult it was to maintain that outward facade!

I didn't know what to do. I was faced with difficult questions: "What about the children? Can I make it alone? I've never had a job. I am uneducated. Who would hire me? Maybe this will blow over"—and on and on.

I realized that I had a choice. I could self-destruct, turning to alcohol or drugs to quiet my broken heart, or I could turn to something that would give me the strength to live through this situation and protect my children and myself from the consequences of my grief. The power of my grief was so overwhelming that it could have destroyed us all.

I had been practicing Yoga for five or six years by that time. I was hardly an expert, but I could not help noticing all the references to Celibacy in some of the books I was reading. I had never felt that that part of Yoga was for me. I was an American, after all, and I believed that my needs and relationships had no connection with those old texts from an Eastern world. But it was true that I was faced not only with the grief of my partner's turning away from me but also with my own sexual needs. I realized that here again I had two choices: to suffer and self-destruct or to transform my experience into something with meaning.

I had to do something, because my constant inner conversation was haunting me. Whenever I tried to rest my mind by getting away from it, it became more furious. I was a complete failure. What saved me was that I could not believe that this was really love and that love could cause me such pain. All my life, I had dreamed of loving and being loved. I refused to blame love for my condition. Actually, my own inborn fantasy of love saved me because it had taken form and refused to die.

Instead of suffering, I decided to try for transformation.

I realized that I really did not know or understand love at

all. I thought that I did, but obviously I was wrong. It was not love's fault that my marriage was falling apart. I decided to get to know love instead of blaming or cursing it. I began to fantasize about the principle of love in a way that allowed the form of love to step away from the emotional, egotistical form that I had given it and take on a form of its own, free of all manipulation—a great, golden form of love alone. In other words, I gave up personal ownership of love.

I did not want to react to my situation like the television melodramas—"Well, if you don't love me, I'll go and find someone who will!"—and in so doing, simply repeat the same old formula of broken hearts that swirls around us all. I decided to stop all mental and physical involvement with sex and love as I had known it and try to get to know and feel and recognize love in ways I had never known before. I began to practice Celibacy. No one ever knew it. It was a totally private affair.

I was following all the same rituals and routines of my life, but my approach was different. At first, I was so lonely. I longed for sex, but the alternatives didn't suit me. So I went to parties as a beginner in the practice of Celibacy, and gradually, I was able to enjoy the beauty of sex in everything around me. The glances, the clothes, the food, the interplay of conversations, even body movement became my classroom of learning new approaches to love. I tried to learn joy in love observed. I tried to feel it in myself.

I had a long talk with myself. Who, I asked, is the person responsible for the only sexual-love relationship in my life? If I am so lonely, who can I ask for relief? I realized that I alone was responsible to know love in my life. No reactionary dependence on anyone else would do. Love was there to be supremely enjoyed, and it was not subject to demand. It was always there, and the choice to enjoy it was totally mine. I was alone with love.

It was obvious to me that I had no ownership of Nature's procreative plan. I was a simple tool in that design. I had tried to call love my own, reveling in its beauty as I liked, and resting on it in a fantasy of thinking that it was always mine and that I had a right to it. This indeed was true. I made my mistake both in demanding that this could be provided for me by someone else and in thinking that it could be removed from me according to someone else's whim—meaning that I could lose love at any time. I had to say to myself, "Wait a minute. Love can't be lost." Instead of continuing long, painful inner conversations with myself about my sadness or loss, I began to practice conversing with love as a separate being.

I began to look for love in everything. I was an observer of sex and love's play, and I saw that love was the unseen support of everything. Love never demands ownership of anything. It exists with or without all our various manipulations. It is the whole show, and it knows it. And Celibacy welcomes you into its presence.

CHAPTER 8

ETHIC #5
NONHOARDING

*Simplify the Things You
Want and Need*

One of the commentaries on Patanjali's *Yoga Sutras*, written by a scholar named Aranya, says this about Nonhoarding (or *Aparigraha* in Sanskrit): "There is trouble in acquiring enjoyables, trouble in preserving them, unhappiness when they're gone." I use this quote because I want to begin by confronting the pervasive and misleading attitudes concerning possessions that permeate many discussions on this topic. The outlook of Yoga is that possessions themselves are not a problem; the difficulty comes in our attitudes toward them—in other words, our feelings of ownership.

In most religious communities, the ability to give up all your material possessions is looked upon as having great merit, because you are told that by doing this you can become closer to God. Eastern traditions respect any person who wears an orange robe and carries a begging bowl, because that person is assumed to be on a spiritual search; therefore, that person deserves and receives support from society. Many people abuse this attitude. Once in India in the early 1970s, I met an American youth who had donned an orange robe simply because, as he put it, "Everyone takes care of you if you wear this. Life here is much easier."

In contrast, in the subtle tradition of Kashmir Shaivism, no special robes are needed to demonstrate the ethic of Nonhoarding. The student works to give up all feelings of ownership for material things, not necessarily the things themselves. (Later in this chapter, I will discuss the problem of ownership of more subtle things, such as relationships and power.) Material things are respected as God's gifts, and so aspirants never denigrate them but maintain the greatest appreciation for all things, considering them to be on loan from God to aid their paths to spirituality. If you were practicing this attitude, you would be neither a spendthrift nor a miser. You would take care of your money and possessions without spending a lot of time thinking about protecting them, increasing them, or being afraid that you will lose them. In the practice of Nonhoarding, you try to remain the same regardless of your possessions.

This attitude is illustrated clearly by the actions of Lakshmanjoo's grandmaster, Rama, and his master, Mahatabkak—both of whom practiced Nonhoarding and were, according to Lakshmanjoo, men who had attained God consciousness.

LAKSHMANJOO: The word *aparigraha* has two parts: "a-" means abandonment; "-parigraha" means collection.

ALICE: Should a student practice Nonhoarding by giving things away, or would it be better to concentrate on a different attitude toward the things that he already has?

LAKSHMANJOO: Thought must not be there of those things.

ALICE: If he needs to use those things, should he keep them? For instance, if the house is full of toys for the children, should he keep the toys? If he has dishes to eat on, should he keep the dishes?

LAKSHMANJOO: Not all the dishes. We have come to the same point again. My grandmaster [Rama] had no *parigraha*. He was practicing *aparigraha*. He had only one *faran* [robe], that is all. If things were presented to him, he put them all in an *almira* [closet]. He didn't touch them, he didn't give them away, he ignored them totally, as if they were not existing at all.

ALICE: Then even giving them away would have shown some connection to the desire of the recipient. And this upset him?

LAKSHMANJOO: Yes. His food was also coming from outside. He didn't cook; he had no kitchen.

ALICE: So he ate whatever was given him?

LAKSHMANJOO: Whatever was carried from one householder. Each morning about sunrise, he would take what he wanted, that's all. No, he didn't worry about the next meal. My master [Mahatabkak] was altogether different; he enjoyed luxuries.

So according to Lakshmanjoo's experience, even a great master can enjoy luxuries. The difference lies in the person's emotional response to these luxuries. We can enjoy everything the world offers if we have the constant realization in the background that "this is not mine; it has been loaned to me for my enjoyment." This type of statement comes from the true ego of the spiritual body. It would not occur to the false ego of the physical body to say this, because it thinks that it owns material things and does not realize where those things actually come from.

ALICE: Doesn't someone who practices Nonhoarding become quite happy?

LAKSHMANJOO: He becomes quite happy, and he has no worry at all.

ALICE: There is no unhappiness in giving up these things because they were never yours, is that true?

LAKSHMANJOO: He does not own them—he's only enjoying them while he's here.

HOW TO BEGIN PRACTICING NONHOARDING

Examine your attitude toward material things. Living and practicing the ethic of Nonhoarding is easy to do with material things. I suggest that you begin this practice by keeping a few beautiful things around you that you enjoy, but do not stuff boxes and closets with what you do not use or need. This does not necessarily mean that you have to have a great deal of wealth at your disposal. I try to make my living quarters as pleasant and attractive as possible because I am happier in that type of atmosphere.

When I lived in the jungle with Rama, our living quarters consisted of a grass hut that was coated on the floor and walls with liquified cow dung. A nice little lady came in twice a week to put a fresh coat on the floor and walls. As it dried, she embellished the whole room with designs and pictures which created an intricate carved pattern. The result was not only beautiful to look at but also very fresh and clean-smelling, like newly mowed hay. My one piece of furniture was a *charpai*, or cot, and I put flowers in water glasses around the room. I was happy there.

Everything depends on where you are and what you have to work with. The main point of Nonhoarding is to not stockpile things you do not use or need. It takes energy to take care of extra belongings—energy that can be put to better use in a more productive way in your life. If you have not used something for a year or more, why not give it to someone who can use it and simplify your living arrangements? Make your living quarters light and free.

Track the discussion in your head. The mental practice of Nonhoarding is a bit more complicated. The key is to give up constant inner conversation about the past. Let the hoarded experiences of the past go gently; do not try to hold on to them. This is a type of hoarding that slows you down and becomes a burden. Do not carry it with you. Try to live in the moment, free and light, unfettered by what has come before. Enjoy spontaneity in your daily life and learn to feel comfortable with new experiences. Enjoy the unexpected. Observe thought patterns in the same way that you clean your closets. If a thought, an idea, or an attitude has not served you for the last year, get rid of it; let it go.

FEAR OF LOSS

Most of us spend a great deal of time worrying about acquiring things, and we worry even more about preserving and protecting them. A great deal of stress is generated by all this anxiety about possessions. Can you see the connection with fear of loss, which we have been talking about throughout this book? It is easy to see that with the practice of Nonhoarding, the fear of loss is annihilated. If you do not own anything, you cannot lose it. Careful, constant observation will show you that all things are provided for you through your spiritual body.

Loss, to most of us, is equated with being vulnerable, humiliated, and impotent. Yet those who are established in Nonhoarding, though they may appear to have nothing, actually have something much more valuable and powerful than ordinary material possessions. In religious communities, for example, the residents generally wear plain clothing and live a simple lifestyle, showing that their attention is given to spiritual rather than physical concerns. The implication is that the real underlying power does not need any outward show.

Aspects of our everyday culture display this attitude as well. Consider the popular minimalist saying of "Less is more," referring to the notion that simplicity is more dynamic than clutter. A similar trend in cooking during the 1980s persuaded us

A LESSON IN OWNERSHIP

The attitude that we can never own anything—not even our own bodies—was illustrated to me very clearly by a story that Lakshmanjoo told me when we were discussing Non-stealing. Several years ago, Lakshmanjoo was walking in the lane near his home when he encountered a Muslim neighbor. Knowing that the Islamic holiday of Ede was in progress, Lakshmanjoo asked the man, "How much meat have you purchased for your feast today?"

The man answered, "I have not purchased any meat. I want meat of human being today."

Lakshmanjoo said, "There is a great Muslim saint living on the other side of the lake; go there and ask for food."

"No," said the neighbor, "he is too old. I want fresh young flesh of saint like you."

Whereupon Lakshmanjoo held out his arm and said, "Then take from my body." At that, the man saluted Lakshmanjoo and walked on.

The idea that nothing belongs to us—not even our own bodies—is difficult to grasp, yet as you continue practicing these ethics, you can eventually begin to realize that consciousness has an existence far beyond the body's limitations.

that a plate overflowing with gaudy calories is less appealing to both body and mind than a few nourishing items artfully arranged. And how many teenagers are proud to drive around in an old and tired-looking car simply because it has a revved-up engine under the hood? In none of these examples is there an idea of deprivation or loss, but rather the opposite: that benefit comes from something other than outward appearances.

In myths and stories around the world, you will read about people who appear in the court of the king in rags, seemingly destitute. But they are greatly respected for their wisdom and power, which have come from their spiritual searches, and this great power surpasses all the material goods that the king and court hold dear.

Because of this legendary belief, in most Asian countries, the king's court is always open to the holy man carrying a begging bowl. The implication is that the spiritual power of that person is more powerful than the kingdom itself. In fact, the holy man represents the source of all power, and all rulers bow to that presence. The simple humility of the holy man, who seems to own nothing, is given the respect of owning every-

THE FLAWED DIAMOND

I remember Rama telling me about a visit he made to a prince in Poona, a city in South India. The family of the prince was suffering from failing harvests and a dwindling fortune. The prince was driving with Rama across a bridge when he pulled a huge diamond out of his coat pocket. It was the size of his hand, and a beautiful image of the goddess Durga riding on her tiger was carved into the center of it.

The prince said, "This has been in our family for generations, and I keep it with me every day to pray to it."

Rama took the diamond out of the prince's hand and said, "But this is no good. There's a crack in it." And he threw it right over his head into the river.

The prince was terribly distraught at the loss of the jewel, and even tried to climb out of the car to retrieve it—but it was lost. Rama comforted him, and, after some time, the family fortunes improved. Because the diamond was cracked, and therefore imperfect, the prayers offered to it also became imperfect. Prayer deserves the very best offering. I always remember this story in connection with Nonhoarding. Rama didn't care at all that it was a huge diamond. He only cared if the offering to God was correct.

> The Yogi to whom a clod of earth, a stone, and a piece of gold make no difference is spoken of as a God-realized soul.
> (The *Bhagavad Gita*)

thing. Gandhi, who wore simple homespun clothes and rope sandals, lived this principle.

Lakshmanjoo spoke to me about a Kashmiri saint who was famous for owning nothing. He had just one loincloth and one cotton shawl. When he saw someone wearing a shawl made of *pashmina* (the most valuable and expensive cloth made from the softest wool of the pashmina goat, which lives high in the Himalayas), he would ask that person to give him the *pashmina*, and he would throw away his cotton shawl. A few days later, he would see someone with a piece of burlap, and he would ask someone to buy that for him and he would throw away the *pashmina* shawl. To him, everything was the same; it was all a gift from God.

OTHER ASPECTS OF OWNERSHIP

The problem of ownership can also be perceived in more subtle "possessions," such as relationships. Lakshmanjoo told me that if you were really attached to someone who died, you would want to die with them. This would mean that you might give up your life without ever knowing the full range of power that lies within your grasp. You would be making a total sacrifice of your future potential. This would be self-destructive, violating the principle of Nonviolence.

Similarly, I have seen many couples hoarding their relationships, spending a lot of time being fearful of what would happen if they were separated instead of using that time to enjoy the happiness of the moment. A possessive attitude, based in false ego, means that you will always be worried about losing what you cannot own. Similar to the ancient king in the old stories of Joseph Campbell's wonderful comparative mythology books, you are chained to a tree with a club in your hand, constantly on guard lest someone come to usurp your position, never able to rest or sleep. This attitude expects the physical body to be responsible for all its cares; it does not allow the spiritual body to enter the picture. The king, on guard against any newcomer, would not be able to recognize the spiritual body when it appears.

The false ego of the physical body fears death, yet the death of the physical body, as the *Gita* says, is an inevitable event. Why not put your efforts into knowing the part of you that never dies? The spiritual body knows no death, and by your knowing the spiritual body, you can also know that.

RESULTS OF PRACTICING NONHOARDING

According to the scholar Patanjali, in his *Yoga Sutras*, the result of practicing Nonhoarding is knowledge of three lives: the life just past, the present life, and the one to come. This may seem like a strange concept, but imagine how you might live if you had the different perspective on life that this would give you. You would realize that this life is not all there is, that you have a much longer time period in which to move toward your goals. This knowledge also would reduce your fear of death.

You might also discover valuable information that would affect the life you are living now. For instance, if you perceive from this phenomenon that you had been a musician in your previous life, it might help you understand your love for music in this one, and you might even learn how to call on past experiences to help you develop your skills.

> ALICE: It would seem that a person who works on becoming established in *Aparigraha* would develop the qualities of generosity and fearlessness. Are there other

qualities that would indicate some progress toward *Aparigraha?*

LAKSHMANJOO: Yes, progress. His spiritual advancement grows very swiftly, without any failure. And his memory is clear for three lives.

ALICE: So, he can see the future, and he can see the present.

LAKSHMANJOO: And he can see the past.

ALICE: And this is very valuable?

LAKSHMANJOO: Yes. His memory for three lives becomes clear because it is not blocked by possessions.

ALICE: So he's not clinging to one thing and being blinded to the other?

LAKSHMANJOO: Yes. He can see whatever is in my past life, what I have to do in this life, and what I will do in next life, after death. He sees. He becomes clairvoyant. This is the fruit of that *Aparigraha.*

This discussion assumes that you are familiar with the idea of reincarnation. In Yoga, as in much of the Eastern world, the belief is that there is more than one life. The spiritual body, which never dies, attaches itself to a succession of physical bodies while the individual works to realize the Universal Body.

I do not encourage my students to brood about what may or may not have occurred in previous lives, or to spend a lot of time speculating on future ones, because until this insight is reached naturally as a result of mastering the ethic of Nonhoarding, it is more useful to concentrate on becoming aware of your present life. I only mention this result because it is described by all the great teachers and because I think that you should know what is possible as a result of practicing these ethics, even if it sounds far-fetched. One of the things that distinguishes Yoga from religion is that in Yoga, you are not expected to believe anything until you experience it yourself.

Lakshmanjoo talked to me once about the importance of Nonhoarding with regard to the powers that are attained as a result of practicing all ten of the ethics. He said that just as one should practice all ethics simultaneously, in the same way, the results of practicing the ethics also will occur simultaneously.

> ALICE: We hear so often of people who abuse and misuse these powers. Can you talk about the responsibility that goes along with this power of attainment?
>
> LAKSHMANJOO: You should neither be excited nor be depressed. If that power is just fading away, don't care. If power is growing too much, don't be excited. Then it remains the same. But power fades away by utilizing it.
>
> ALICE: In other words, it is not yours to use. It has its own plan for what it will do.
>
> LAKSHMANJOO: Yes.

This discussion about power with my great teacher puzzled me at first because, as an American, I believed that if I was practicing and learning how to be powerful, one of the greatest joys would be to use it and feel it. Our culture greatly values power of all kinds. Business deals often depend on the person who wields the greatest power in the marketplace, and the seduction of political power probably drives most political campaigns. Some of the most successful films have to do with the attainment of power and its use for good or evil. A prime example is the *Godfather* series.

This view of power is entirely opposite to the ethical principle of Nonhoarding because all power, in fact, comes from the spiritual body. The attempted manipulation of power by the false ego of the physical body will always end in grief since the false ego has only a limited perspective.

I have seen this happen many times in interactions between parents and children. Once, a thirteen-year-old girl was listening to the radio and dreamily announced to her mother, "I want to be a singer when I grow up." Her mother immediately replied with what she considered a practical response: "Oh, you don't have that kind of voice." The girl never mentioned it

THE SORCERER'S APPRENTICE

The fairy tale of the sorcerer's apprentice illustrates the misplaced use of power. The apprentice desired more than anything to have the power his master exhibited, but he saw only the outward manifestation of that power, not where it came from or how to use it wisely. One night, after the sorcerer had gone to sleep, the apprentice stole his master's wand and repeated a spell. Chaos ensued until the master woke and was able to put things right. The apprentice had succeeded in briefly wielding power, but he did not know how to control it.

again and in the future was less inclined to confide her hopes and dreams to her mother. The mother's false ego had leaped to a completely unnecessary judgment, a use of power that violated the ethical principle of Nonviolence and blocked the freedom of the child's fantasy, which could be a picture of her future growth.

Our best interests are served by stepping aside and inviting the spiritual body to use the power that comes from ethical practice without interference from the physical body. In the example above, if the mother had waited for input from her spiritual body before responding, she probably would have replied with encouragement rather than with disparagement and kept the channels of relationship open and free with her child.

My attitude about power started to change when I began to practice meditation, because in that state where my breath stopped and my mind became silent, I came to know that something else was running the show besides my physical body. I felt no panic. I was quite comfortable, and I was aware of great support and power coming to me from within.

I no longer thought that my physical body had to keep me alive, and I no longer thought that my physical body owned my life. I gave up that idea, and in so doing, the channel between my physical and spiritual bodies opened and power flowed into me easily. Once I experienced this sense of power coming from my spiritual body, I realized I could choose to move between my physical and spiritual consciousness at will. It was a new flexibility of thought and it brought me great happiness. All separateness was gone. I had joined my outer self with my inner self.

CHAPTER 9

ETHIC #6
PURITY

Make Yourself Clear and Powerful

The ethic of Purity (or *Shauch*, in Sanskrit) is essentially about being 100 percent yourself: unfragmented, strong, and confident. Most of us present different faces to different people. We say one thing and do another, and we are not always clear about who we are or the direction of our lives.

This fragmentation keeps us from becoming as powerful as we could be. For instance, you cannot become a concert pianist if you practice the piano only a half-hour per day. In order to become a superb pianist, your whole life must be dedicated to it. Even when you are not actually at the piano, you are thinking about the music, planning your concert schedule, and preparing yourself in many different ways, all centered on becoming an exceptional pianist.

The practice of Purity teaches you how to reduce the quality of separateness in life so that you can focus on what you want and make a determined effort to achieve it. This takes the participation of both bodies:

THE POWER OF BEING YOURSELF

Throughout my career as a Yoga teacher, I have worked with many students who were troubled by frequent anxiety attacks, during which they felt fractured and powerless. In all cases, I discovered that these feelings emerged because these students had no concept of who they were or what they wanted to do with their lives. There was no clear effort to reach any goal, and so there was no chance for any goal to take shape.

Consider people who have had a strong influence on the world, such as Gandhi, Mother Teresa, or Albert Einstein. Even though their goals were widely varied, all of them had one thing in common: They were intently focused on what they perceived as their purpose in life. A clear vision of their goals gave them strength. They were practicing a type of Purity in body, mind, and speech because everything they did, thought, or said was dedicated to what they believed in.

physical and spiritual. Purity clears the channel between the two bodies so they can work together in strength and power.

HOW TO BEGIN PRACTICING PURITY

Yogic texts describe three domains in which to practice Purity: body, mind, and speech.

Make your body as healthy as possible. Purity of the body includes physical cleanliness and clean, beautiful surroundings. Yoga exercises and breathing techniques can help a great deal to maintain optimum health and strength. Breathing techniques are especially helpful because they make your nervous system strong enough to handle the extra energy generated as your spiritual body begins to emerge.

LAKSHMANJOO: There is one element in body that is the purest. That is breath. Purest element in body is breath. And through breath, you can reach God.

ALICE: Does this Purity of the body bring about a cessation of the fear of death?

LAKSHMANJOO: Yes.

Keeping your body strong, healthy, and clean is a natural starting point for Purity because you are inviting the spiritual body to join with you, and, as a good host, you want your environment to be as welcoming as possible. A conversation begins in your mind, directed toward the spiritual body: "I am trying to coax you to come forth in all your beauty. I am trying to make myself something you would love to join with." It's a seduction of your spiritual self, and you're trying everything you can think of to persuade it to appear. You make yourself beautiful, thinking, "Do you like these clothes? Is this color pleasing?"

Your conversation extends to all the food you eat. You are essentially eating for two, and you want the food you give that growing spiritual body to be as pure as you can make it. It becomes an enchanting game: "Do you like this? Would you prefer that?" And in the end, you are eating and drinking intuitively. Fasting for the sake of Purity would be impossible. One does not starve the physical body when it is trying to coax the spiritual body to join with it. The result would be disastrous: As you starve the physical body into a weak state, the spiritual body has to carry the whole load. This never works. The spiritual body will retreat if the physical is not strong enough to carry its share.

Now widen this outlook a bit and consider everything else that you "eat" through your other senses. A careful mental diet is necessary to clean and strengthen the mind. This is not a religious proscription against violent movies, loud music, and so on. The point is, how do the things you watch, listen to, smell, and touch affect your thoughts and feelings? How do you react? Do you enjoy the reaction? How long does the reaction stay with you? A student of ethics tries always to observe and make choices based on these observations—not on those that are someone else's opinion. It takes constant alertness in order to remain steady in the face of multiple distractions.

Protect your mind against fragmentation. Purity of mind has been described as "not being disturbed by a myriad of thoughts." One of the easiest ways to practice mental Purity is to simply observe your thoughts without judgment or censure. This will automatically detach you slightly from upset or discomfort associated with your thoughts.

Lakshmanjoo says in one of his books that when you are walking, for instance, you perceive all the features of the landscape, such as the grass, the trees, and the clouds, but they don't leave impressions on your mind. He recommends acting in the world in the same way: Do everything but leave the impressions behind. In Shaivism, you are taught to simply observe, and then move on. Do not let the impression bind you.

You do this by learning to tolerate the pairs of opposites (such as pain and pleasure, cold and hot, happy and sad, angry and loving) so they leave no impression. When opposites no longer cause an imbalance and you rest comfortably between them, in the center position, you feel connected to all existence. When this occurs, all experience of separateness is gone.

Speak carefully and truthfully. Purity of speech refers to speech that is true to yourself and which does not harm anyone. When your speech matches your inner thoughts and feelings, you are practicing Purity of speech. Young children naturally display this quality. They say exactly what they are feeling. They have not yet learned how to be deceptive, so they express themselves purely. Sophistication, which our adult culture values so highly, is attained by piling layer upon layer of false representation.

In this sense, Purity of speech implies a certain assertiveness that comes from the confidence of knowing that your physical and spiritual bodies are operating in concert. When practicing Purity of speech, you would not speak deceitfully or

THE POWER TO CHOOSE

As I was sitting for my lessons with Lakshmanjoo one day in Kashmir, I noticed that he was obviously uncomfortable with toothache. I felt sad that he was in pain and told him so. He replied, "Oh, I don't waste energy on that. I have two choices: I can hate it or I can enjoy it. I am choosing to enjoy it." The power to choose between suffering and enjoyment in such a situation, I believe, is a tremendous gift that all of us would be grateful for.

carelessly. You would not say one thing and do another. When your inner and outer thoughts match, this Purity gives you supreme poise and great strength of purpose.

Bringing body, mind, and speech together in harmony results in Purity, which unites the two bodies in a solid body of power. It is exactly similar to the way great athletes prepare for a contest. They use everything at their disposal to reach for their goals of peak performance. Their intense physical and mental preparations are one-pointed; the same intense preparation is needed when practicing ethical behavior.

USE OPPOSITES TO REACH THE CENTER

Start by simply observing all thought and feeling in terms of opposites. For example, you hear an old song on the radio and it reminds you of some tender experience. The music rides on the vehicle of remembrance of emotion. Pay full attention to the feeling that the music evokes in you. Then consciously move to the opposite feeling. If the song evoked sadness in you, consciously feel joyful. If the song excites you, feel as you would if it were a lullaby. This practice shows you that you are the same in both cases. You are moving from one emotion to another only by choice.

Now take the exercise one step further: Imagine the song playing as before, but try to have no reaction of any kind. Choose to be absolutely still and aware in the center, between the opposites. That is the practice of Purity. You are aware of both feelings, instead of becoming stuck on one type of feeling only. This will help you become less fragmented.

A student who was practicing this exercise wrote to me about her experiences.

I was confused about my feelings for a man I was seeing, so I tried this exercise of working with opposites. I started with how I was feeling in the present and labeled this extreme Choice A—I stated it as a desire: "I want a man who is mean, self-absorbed, unavailable when I need him, afraid of intimacy, and who devalues my life." Then I stated the opposite, Choice B: "I want a man who deeply cares about me, values my life, supports me, loves me, and is around when I need him."

I went back and forth between the two sides, and I don't know how it happened, but I realized that my unhappy feelings were not the fault of this man; they were a choice I was making. Even though I cared very much about this person, I was in a relationship that I didn't want. This exercise of seeing things in terms of opposites cracked my emotional shell and things started to unravel for me. I didn't know how to turn my back on a relationship when I had such strong feelings for a person, but after seeing the situation, I couldn't go on the way I had been, hoping and waiting for things to change.

The next morning, I woke with an incredible sense of loss. I cried all day. I felt there was no way to go for what I wanted without losing what I had. I sat down and wrote him a letter stating what I wanted, and it was simple and clear. I don't know the results yet, but I've made a decision to live by it.

I was so struck by the light that this exercise shed on my muddled thinking and the effect it had in helping me clearly see what I wanted in a relationship. Of course, no one wants Choice A, as I stated it above, and who wouldn't want Choice B? Yet the situation had evolved into Choice A without my realizing it. It occurred to me that I have spent a great deal of my life like this: not knowing exactly what I wanted, so hanging on to what I had and not letting it go even if I wasn't happy. And how could I see what I wanted when I was so busy hanging on to what I had and trying to form it into something it wasn't?

I have tried this exercise several times over the past few days. In each case, when I'm unhappy about something, I state the present feeling as a choice: "I want . . . . " Then I state the opposite. I never want Choice A. Yet time and again, I find myself there. This exercise is a great tool for making my choices very conscious and successful.

BREAK THE PATTERN OF ADDICTIVE THOUGHT

Meditation is another way to practice mental Purity. Meditation helps break the pattern of what I call addictive thought, an example of fragmented thinking. Addictive thought means being stuck in one way of thinking about something, such as believing that every discussion with your boss will turn out badly for you.

Meditation, which is simply practicing not thinking about anything for a period of time, teaches you how to rest in the center, between two opposite thoughts, giving your spiritual body a chance to speak. (See page 136 for a brief description of how to begin meditating.) The more you do this, the more you will be able to break addictive thought patterns by seeing other possibilities. Meditation gives you a glimpse into that state where the spiritual body and the physical body are one.

PURITY

"Blessed are the pure in heart, for they shall see God."
This well-known line from the Bible illustrates the power of
Purity. Those who are "pure in heart" are balanced between
opposites. Because they are not fragmented, the channel between their physical and spiritual bodies is clear. They see
no separateness between themselves and anyone or anything else, and no separateness between themselves and
God. Therefore, God, their spiritual body, is always available to them.

RESULTS OF PRACTICING
PURITY

Purity of body, mind, and speech helps heal the separateness that we all feel from time to time. The longing for an end
to separateness is a constant theme in Western literature, especially in writings about utopias. The goal of wholeness seems
vague and unreachable, but if you practice the ethic of Purity,
wholeness is within your grasp. You no longer feel diluted, fragmented, or split, and you feel connected with your spiritual self.

Another wonderful result of practicing Purity is the development of what I call peripheral awareness: the ability to see
beyond your immediate reactions and perceptions that emanate
from only the physical body.

Lakshmanjoo once commented to me, "Doesn't that bird's
song taste delicious?" How could he taste the song of the bird?
Very simply, he was not bound to only one way of perceiving
the bird's song because his spiritual body was functioning as
clearly as his physical body. Some people naturally experience
this type of crossover of the senses, called synesthesia, but the
type of intuitive experience that springs from the spiritual body
is different and is available to anyone with practice.

Peripheral awareness means that you can become completely aware of everything. You can notice every thought, every reaction, every feeling—and then have the ability to move away from involvement to clear observation. This ability will complement the practice outlined above when you observe that you are stuck in opposites, because peripheral awareness shows you that you have other choices. Lakshmanjoo described this state of peripheral awareness by saying that it is important to maintain awareness that is neither external awareness nor internal awareness, but rather the center of the deepest aspects of these two. He called this the most refined type of awareness. The center position, the middle state between opposites, is where Purity is found.

PRACTICING PERIPHERAL AWARENESS

You've been asked to attend a cocktail party connected with your business. When you arrive, you realize that you don't see anyone you know. At first, you feel nervous and upset, and this prevents you from seeing much around you, because all your attention is focused on your anxious feelings. Then you remember the ethic of Purity. You call up a feeling opposite to anxiety, such as comfort or enjoyment, and this helps you to lessen your initial feelings of discomfort as you move toward the middle position, between the two opposite feelings.

When your anxiety lessens, you are able to look around you, sensing where you will be comfortable and having the needed poise to present yourself and your work. You will have more confidence as you begin to talk with people, knowing that you are able to project your true self.

CHAPTER 10

ETHIC #7
CONTENTMENT

Practice Being Happy in the Moment

The common meaning for the word "content-ment" is satisfaction with what one has. In Yogic ethics, however, the practice of Con-tentment (*Santosh* in Sanskrit) is not connected with an emotion, but rather with a state of consciousness. It is best described as the ability to remain in the present moment.

One day, when I did not have to go anywhere or do anything, I decided that I would practice the ethic of Contentment. To do this, I told myself that I would not think of anything in the past—any remembrance of any kind—and I would not think or plan or hope for anything in the future. I sat quietly in my meditation pose and absolutely refused to allow my mind to move backward or forward. I held it firmly in the middle.

After a few minutes of this intense focus, I found it very difficult to move. It took great effort to straighten

More and more, I'm happy in myself. I'm aware of a great silent strength like the inner core of myself. Sometimes it's distinctly there. Sometimes I am aware of it dimly in the background. (An excerpt from a student's letter)

out my legs and arms, and I had no impulse to stand or move in any direction. I felt exactly as if I had stepped into a swamp, where every step was difficult. It was as if my physical body was echoing my mental exercise by becoming reluctant to move in any direction. The feeling of being practically immobile overcame me.

Then I became overwhelmed by a giddy sensation of freedom. I found myself freely floating in a mystical state of detachment where I could clearly observe what was happening around me without becoming involved. A golden feeling of strength was supporting me. I cannot describe it in words, but I remember it now, even though I have moved out of that state.

It may seem, from my story, that practicing Contentment in this way would turn you into a useless lump, unable to support your life or work. But what I have found is that by practicing this exercise, I am able to welcome a totally new source of support and power from my spiritual body. My experience helped me discover that Contentment is part of the spiritual body. I was able to feel its support when my physical body became quiet. Though previously unrecognized, this support had always been within my grasp; it was only waiting for me to become aware enough to clear the channel to my spiritual body. That is exactly what the books on Yoga say happens when the spiritual body begins to emerge.

How is it possible, or even desirable, to not think of the past or the future, you ask? Well, I discovered that my hopes and dreams for the future, and the poignancy of the past, were taking up most of my time. In practicing this exercise, I realized that I had missed great delights in the present while I

THE POWER OF CONTENTMENT

A long time ago, during my months of training in India with Rama, I accompanied him on a very difficult lecture tour from Delhi to Dharwar, hundreds of miles to the south. When we finally got back to Delhi, we were exhausted, and a kind devotee of Rama offered us the use of his car to drive to Rama's home in the jungle above Haridwar. I didn't realize what a sacrifice this was at the time. Cars were so precious in India, and besides, I, a woman, would be driving since Rama did not know how. This was soon after the British had left India, and women drivers were unusual.

In my American way, I asked if we had a spare tire and whether the car had been checked out for the long trip. I was assured that all was okay, and in my ignorance, I believed them. We left Delhi in the late afternoon. Rama read the road signs for me, and we progressed well on our way.

Night fell and we slowed down in the intense darkness. We crawled along, among heavily wooded, lonely areas of the jungle. As we stopped in a clearing to check our direction, a tire exploded. I opened the trunk to get out the spare and found it flat and damaged. I was extremely frightened.

Being stranded in these places at night is no joke. I feared for our lives. Rama, however, did not. He pointed out the beauty of the moon. He offered me some water and sat down with me to enjoy the evening. He leaned back on his hands—I can see him now—and said, looking at the sky, "You know, Alice, it's a lovely night." I couldn't say much.

After about twenty minutes, we heard a bell in the distance. Then a man on a bicycle rode into our clearing. He said that he was on his way home from work—he was a mechanic—and he just happened to have his toolbox with him on the back of the bike. He proceeded to change and repair both tires and refused all payment, saying that God had sent him on this path to serve and he was fortunate to have found us. We went on our way in the night. I was very quiet.

wandered in the past or future. The state of consciousness referred to in Shaivism as wonder, delight, and astonishment is a simple description of something wonderful that we have not known before: the joy of the present moment. According to Shaivism, the ethic of contentment can only manifest in the present moment, never in the future or past. If we can pay attention to the present moment in our lives, it can bring great happiness because our attention does not become confused with past experience, nor does it take second place to the hopes for the future.

HOW TO BEGIN PRACTICING CONTENTMENT

Practice resting in the present moment. Simply sit quietly and observe your inner conversation. Each time you notice your thoughts moving to the past or the future, gently bring your attention back to the present moment. It may help to close your eyes. This is an excellent exercise to try in situations where you have to wait for several minutes, such as in a doctor's office, but I would not recommend trying this in your car waiting for traffic to move along.

Try practicing meditation. In meditation, you quiet your mind and body fully, bring your awareness to your forehead, and try to stop all inner conversation. All desires and all thought processes eventually stop, or at least slow down. You no longer feel desire as a whip. The feeling you will experience in meditation is very similar to the feeling you experience when you are stable in the ethic of Contentment.

To get the most out of meditative practice, make sure that you will not be disturbed for ten to fifteen minutes. Sit or lie with your back, neck, and head in a straight line. Wear loose, comfortable clothes. Keep yourself warm. (For a more complete description of how to meditate, see the Resources section on page 189 for beginning Yoga manuals.)

Repeat a mantram. The restful space of the present moment is encouraged by Yogis with the constant repetition of a mantram—a special sound formula. If you don't have a specific mantram given to you by a qualified teacher, use the mantram "Om." Use the repetition of this sound to help you stop your inner conversation and rest in the present moment. This can be done silently or aloud. Try this technique any time of day to help bring your attention back to the present. Be sure to take time periodically to notice how the exercise is affecting you.

CONTENTMENT AND DESIRE

Desire is the opposite of Contentment. It is the mechanism that constantly moves our attention either backward to the past, in wanting to repeat some happy experience, or forward, to dwell upon future wants and dreams. Desire avoids the middle state where Contentment lies.

Desire feeds the constant inner conversation of the mind that makes it so difficult to focus on the present. You may not realize how much of your inner conversation is taken up by the effect of desire. For example, remember the last time you heard a beautiful song that stirred your memory. Your attention immediately moved backward to re-experience the event associated with the song. Or think of walking past a store window and seeing something you like; you may begin to imagine yourself wearing or using that thing some time in the future.

Desire always has to do with what is known. If you can articulate a desire for a new car, for instance, you can usually picture what type of car it would be and imagine yourself driving around in it. In the same way, when you call up a memory, let's say, a favorite pet from your childhood, you can be reasonably sure that you are remembering correctly. All these are things you already know.

Contentment, however, lies in the middle of these two extremes of future desire and past memory. In Contentment lies nothing you have known before, but something new, astonishing, and wonderful, because when you practice Contentment, you invite your spiritual body to speak to you, and its voice is spontaneous, unexpected, and unique.

If you let your mind simply wander in the past or the future, never stopping in the present, it is similar to being strapped to a treadmill, going nowhere and never being able to break out of its pattern. Past and future are based in fantasy.

Consider the parable told by Plato, about a man who had lived all his life in a cave. One day, he ventured out into the sunlight, yearning to be free from the confines of the cave, but he couldn't stand the bright light and heat and ran back into the familiar cave, determined never to leave again. This describes so many of us. Like the man in the cave, we fear any change in our perception. We continue behaving in a familiar way, because it is the only way we know. We cling to memory (past) and desire (future) because we do not want our fantasy of the past or future disturbed or changed.

The way to break out of this pattern is to carefully put your inner conversation to rest for a few minutes at a time, as I did in my exercise. Do not go forward in planning, nor backward in memory. Take the position in the middle where there is no thought, no conversation, and no movement at all. Gently stop all thought. Refuse to go forward or backward. Wait and observe in silence.

The first time that you will become aware of the spiritual body is that point of Contentment where you rest in the middle position, perfectly balanced between future and past. The great joy of Contentment is the expression of the spiritual body that is now able to speak. The silence that you have provided in your mind opens the passageway between the two bodies.

Contentment is not the same as endurance of life's various conditions. Many of us are subject to unpleasant and demanding factors in our lives, and most of us learn to live with that awareness. Sometimes we even forget that they are not what we would have chosen and simply take them in stride. This cannot be confused with Contentment as it is described in Shaivite literature. Contentment gives you the ability to be comfortable and happy wherever you are, in all circumstances. Past and future are stilled, and you can have full enjoyment in the moment.

I have tried throughout this book to emphasize the fact that these ethics cannot be understood intellectually. Describing Contentment intellectually, you might say, "I feel content," in other words, using an adjectival form. An intellectual, adjectival approach is always based in the physical body. The spiritual body, however, deals in nouns. Here is one way to picture this concept.

Future is unborn, past is dead. You have to live in present. (Lakshmanjoo, who lived this principle daily. Even as insurrection was tearing his city apart, he spent most of each day working in his beautiful garden.)

Try to fantasize Contentment as an actual form, a bubble perhaps, with you totally protected inside its flexible walls, shimmering among space, supplied with its own power and direction, like a spaceship. The actual form and force are parts of the spiritual body. The ethical student tries to become part of that body to experience its form.

Lakshmanjoo says that a person can be content only if he will. In other words, a person has to consciously seek Contentment. The practice of Contentment calls for self-control and tolerance. It is a difficult balance of indulging a little bit in everything, but not becoming a glutton about anything. Gluttony, or desire, prevents the mind from remaining alert. Without such alertness, you cannot maintain the proper strength of concentration.

Self-control is a harsh word to Westerners—a lot like celibacy—because it implies that a prison of restraint has been put upon you so you cannot do what you want to do. It is a feeling of not being free. But used correctly, without violence, self-control can make you extremely powerful in your ability to enjoy and direct your life. As you progress to fulfilling yourself as a strong individual, self-control becomes a much-loved addition to your everyday activities. You can direct yourself successfully to what you want, and you become very proud of yourself.

DEALING WITH LOSS

The state of Contentment seems to be most difficult to reach at a time of loss or grief, when it is hard to think about anything else. Almost all of us suffer these feelings at some time in our lives, whether it is the death of a child or other loved one, the grief of a divorce, or the grief of illness.

We experience loss every day. The strong individual hopes that whatever happens can be endured with poise and balance, and Contentment can help you attain this. I believe that some regular training in ethics, especially the practice of Contentment, can greatly affect the way you handle all your relationships.

Consider how you feel when someone you love dies. When you are experiencing severe grief, your mind refuses to stay in the moment. It constantly goes either to the past, reliving precious memories, or to the future, dreading life without that person. If you try practicing Contentment, bringing your mind to a middle position in the present moment, it will help to ease the feeling of loss. This is because you are opening the channel to your spiritual body, which can give you the support you need at this time. The strength of your spiritual body will help you replace the loss.

RESULTS OF PRACTICING CONTENTMENT

According to some great mystics, becoming established in Contentment is considered to be one of the greatest jewels of

A STORY ABOUT MAYA

In a popular tale from Indian mythology, the sage Narada played and sang for the god Vishnu, pleasing him so much that Vishnu said, "Ask me for whatever you wish." Narada replied, "I wish to know the secret of Maya." Maya is a word that describes the veil that covers the true reality of the world.

Vishnu said, "Oh, that is very difficult to understand. Choose something else." But Narada insisted, so Vishnu finally said, "All right, go to the village and get me some water to drink, and then I will tell you."

So Narada went to the village and stopped at the headmaster's home. The headmaster's beautiful daughter answered his greeting, and Narada temporarily forgot himself in contemplating her beauty. Then he remembered to ask for water. While she was getting it, the headmaster came out, greeted Narada, and offered him some refreshment. Since they were both interested in spiritual matters, they began talking, and soon evening came. The headmaster invited Narada to spend the night, saying that it would be too hard to find his way back in the dark. Narada accepted.

The next morning, the headmaster asked Narada's advice about village matters and took him on a tour of the village. Gradually, Narada forgot why he had come to the village in the first place. After some time, he married the daughter, had two lovely children, and took over the running of the village.

One summer, a particularly fierce monsoon came, and floodwaters poured through the village. In attempting to escape with his family, Narada lost everything and was himself swept away by the roiling waters. He hit his head on a tree branch and lost consciousness. He awoke to find himself lying under the tree where he had left Vishnu, who was gently saying, "Narada, where is my water? I have been waiting half an hour."

attainment by a human being. The result of this practice is stated in the classic texts of Kashmir Shaivism: "The fruit that accrues from mastering Contentment is that you become completely at peace in this lifetime." When you are able to dwell easily in the present, the stress of rehashing past events or dreading future ones simply falls away.

Lakshmanjoo very clearly said to me that when you move your mind to the middle unmoving position between the opposites of future and past, you are totally supported by your divine self—in other words, by your spiritual body. To me, then, Contentment means being free from thoughts that distract me from the union with myself.

CHAPTER 11

ETHIC #8
TOLERANCE

Encourage Heroic Capability in Yourself

The Sanskrit word for this ethic, *Tapas*, is sometimes translated as "heat," a meaning that is associated with cleansing or purifying. Metals, for example, are refined, or purified, by application of intense heat. With regard to Yoga, the heat of *Tapas* refers to the purification of the physical nature. Yogic exercises and breathing techniques turn up your body's thermostat, purifying the physical nature with heat so that it can tolerate the extra energy produced by the emergence of the spiritual body. Energy produced in this way is often described as a bright inner fire.

When Lakshmanjoo talked about *Tapas*, he used the word Tolerance, and that is the meaning I will use throughout this chapter. Tolerance is an important characteristic of a hero. Heroic capability means more than the ordinary ability to withstand life's pressures with steadiness, perseverance, and courage. A hero

THE HEAT OF TOLERANCE

I experienced a strong heat reaction in the early years of my practice. My body became so hot that I began swimming in Lake Erie while the spring ice was still in the water. I would wrap wet sheets around me to cool me, and the heat was so intense that it would dry the sheets. This condition lasted for about five years. Lakshmanjoo told me that Yogis prefer living high in the Himalayas because it is cold. The periods of heat bloom and subside as the second nervous system begins to take shape along with the spiritual body.

stands out as a leader, someone who is not afraid to take up the search for meaning in life, someone who recognizes the constant support of the spiritual body and is able to call on this extra support whenever it is needed.

ALICE: I remember a saying about Swiss mountaineers: "A hero is a man who can stand one minute more." Would you say that describes *Tapas* in any way?

LAKSHMANJOO: That is *Tapas*.

The term *Tapas* is often translated as discipline, or austerity, words that have harsh and unpleasant connotations. Many people believe that painful or difficult practices are necessary for spiritual growth—or even physical fitness, as in the phrase "No pain, no gain." It is important to state that my use of the word Tolerance does not imply suffering. Yoga is not a harsh physical endurance test. Harshness to the body would violate the ethic of Nonviolence (see chapter 4). Tolerance grows with happy practice, and you will enjoy feeling the new strength that this practice supplies as you become comfortable with a new flexibility in your personality and your body. As with all the ethical states, it becomes a resting place, strong and secure.

ALICE: What kind of attitude should a beginning student have in order to be successful in practicing Tolerance?

LAKSHMANJOO: It must be maintained secretly. It must not be exposed. He has to practice it every day. And he has not to show it. You become example of *Tapas*, and you have to live in it, that is all; you have not to preach. Renunciation is not the point. The point is just to live in that. You have not to renounce.

ALICE: So then *Tapas* is not denial, is it? It's not giving anything up; it's choosing how you are going to live.

LAKSHMANJOO: Yes, your behavior. Soothing behavior, it must not be harsh. You must live that way. You have to live that way; you have not to teach that way.

ALICE: Yes. So all this suffering in the name of God certainly has nothing to do with *Tapas*, has it? These people who beat themselves with bramble bushes and stand in the Ganges with their arms held up until they wither away is not *Tapas*, is it?

LAKSHMANJOO: No, it is not *Tapas*. It is just to collect money. If you don't go to office, you have to do something. You go to the river and stand and make money.

ALICE: In mythology, there are many stories about people doing austerities in order to get the attention of God or gain some power. Is this a proper use of *Tapas*?

LAKSHMANJOO: No, this is not proper. There must not be a show.

HOW TO BEGIN PRACTICING TOLERANCE

Transform your outlook on mundane tasks. Any task, provided it does not cause violence to anyone or anything, can be used to practice Tolerance. You can easily begin to practice Tolerance in your work, your family life, and other daily activities. Consider the mundane daily task of cleaning the kitchen after a meal—a job that most people prefer to avoid. Take on this work happily as an exercise in Tolerance.

The way to make this daily task a happy one is to give it meaning for you. You will gain great respect for the work as well as pride in yourself because you have proven that you can make this small effort regularly and competently, without complaint. The size of the task is not important; what matters is the flexible, steady attitude that you are developing by making and keeping a commitment.

When I first practiced Yoga, I would deliberately choose the most monotonous tasks, such as shelling peas and packing them in quart jars or hemming large tablecloths by hand. As I worked, I was able to transform my outlook about any job so that I did not merely endure it but instead began to enjoy it. Tolerance helped me to find pleasure in long, tedious hours because I was learning to respect my ability to complete the task.

Many times I have heard students equate patience with Tolerance. They are not the same at all. Patience has to do with remaining in the present moment (see chapter 10). Developing the quality of patience helps you stay in the present moment, rather than leaping ahead to when the job is done. This characteristic of present-moment awareness helps you build steadiness, one of the heroic qualities of Tolerance.

Observe the other nine ethics daily. All ten ethical principles are interconnected. I've mentioned several times in this book how Nonviolence, for instance, is a foundation for every other ethic. Tolerance has a similarly broad application. The greatest practice of Tolerance is constant attention to *all* the ethical principles. By giving yourself the task of examining every action and thought in the light of ethics, such as Nonviolence, Truthfulness, and Nonstealing, you develop the courage to change and the perseverance to keep on trying day after day.

These are the qualities of a hero in tune with the spiritual body. It is a happy challenge to become more flexible, discovering that you are doing all of this for yourself. You gain pride in the person that you are becoming.

Practice breathing techniques. Yogic breathing exercises can help develop Tolerance by increasing the heat in the body. This increased heat will cleanse your nervous system, contributing to better health and revealing a new sensitivity to yourself and your world. There is no need to attempt vigorous advanced breathing techniques, which can be dangerous if done without proper supervision. The best breathing techniques are gentle exercises such as the Complete Breath, described below.

Begin by sitting on the edge of a chair so your back is straight. Tuck your feet under the chair so your hips are higher than your knees. This will keep your lower back from getting tired. You can also practice this technique lying flat on the floor or on your bed, but do not put a pillow under your head. If you would like to sit cross-legged on the floor, sit on a firm cushion to raise your hips and release tension in your lower back.

Place your hands on your belly and breathe out through your nose. Feel your stomach muscles tightening to push all the air out. Now release your stomach muscles and feel the air start to come in. Continue inhaling, expanding your stomach, your ribs, and your chest, until you are full. Then slowly start to breathe out in reverse, letting your chest relax first, then your ribs, and finally, tightening your stomach as before to complete the exhalation.

Repeat five to ten times. Try to make the inhalation and exhalation approximately equal in length, and breathe as slowly as you can without strain. Always breathe through your nose. Concentrate on the sound of the breath.

Besides helping to increase Tolerance, this exercise will improve concentration and help you reduce anxiety, stress, depression, and insomnia.

Use fantasy. I have often employed a fantasy exercise to encourage students to practice Tolerance. Most of us have been taught that fantasy can never be real and therefore it can never have a real connection with our lives—it remains a dream. I have discovered that directed fantasy can help students approach change. Fantasy helps you to visualize change before it happens, and the ability to welcome change is one of the heroic qualities of Tolerance.

Start this fantasy exercise by lying down in a comfortable position with your eyes closed, or sit straight and relaxed in a chair. Take a few deep breaths through your nose. Let your face relax. Drop your collarbones toward the floor and relax them. Let your hands lie palms up with fingers limp. Relax your hips and your legs, your feet and your back. Get very comfortable, very quiet.

Imagine that you are standing at one end of a long hallway. Visualize something you have always wanted, and place it at the end of the hall. Imagine everything about it in minute detail. Give yourself a moment or two to completely visualize this object of your desire at the end of the hall.

Now pretend that an adversary has come between you and your desired object in the hallway. You can still see your desired object, but when this adversary suddenly appears and stands between you and your goal, it blocks your approach. What is happening? Who or what is your adversary?

Observe this scene carefully for a minute or two.

Now, very slowly let the fantasy picture dissolve. Take a deep breath, open your eyes, and carefully review what has happened in your fantasy.

Most people who truly desire to change have trouble recognizing the stumbling blocks in their way. This exercise shows you what is keeping you from your goal by giving it a form. You will find that this technique is very helpful if you are fighting an addiction. It is difficult to see what urges you to drink or take drugs or smoke, and this exercise gives that urge a form. When you see it, you will be able to deal with it in a different way.

Many students have been greatly helped by practicing this fantasy technique. I would like to share with you a few letters from students about their experiences.

My adversary started out as a big black knight on a big black horse and then it got very nebulous, just a big black thing. I was still trying to figure out how to trick it and get around it when you ended the exercise. It did cross my mind that the adversary came out of me.

• • •

I saw the adversary step in, and I could still see what I wanted at the end of the hall, but I felt powerless to confront the adversary to get what I wanted.

• • •

The first time I tried the fantasy exercise of seeing myself as I wanted to be at the end of the hall, I was unable to see anything for a long time. There did not seem to be any adversary in front of me. Later, I realized that my inability to visualize myself the way I want to be was in itself the adversary.

• • •

I started visualizing the person I'd always wanted to be. Nothing appeared to stop me from moving toward it. But then there was a real feeling of fear in me. And I asked myself, why am I afraid? And where does this come from? And then all of a sudden, I heard this voice saying, "Don't do that. You really don't want that. Stay back. Stay back." It wasn't my voice. It was my aunt's [his guardian's] voice.

Whether you are using this technique to overcome an addiction, to bring about some other needed change in your life, or to bring your spiritual nature into bloom, you will find that it is easier to deal with a form than with something unseen. Form gives you something to work with.

RESULTS OF PRACTICING TOLERANCE

The practice of Tolerance causes an internal transformation that shows outwardly as a greater flexibility and a steadiness in the personality. Although upsets in life still occur, their results are not so devastating because you are aware of the support of your spiritual body and you know that you are not alone. You will especially notice a much greater flexibility in your relationships.

I have noticed this change in my students in many ways. A very mundane example is the student whose outlook was so rigid that she became very upset if her partner did not load the dishwasher according to the manual. After practicing Tolerance for some time, her flexibility increased so much that she was able to enjoy the diversity of options regarding dishwasher loading for the first time.

Another student had to deal with a lifelong inability to disagree with those he loved. When his wife's mother moved into the couple's small apartment after a stroke and required constant care, he was greatly stressed by his lack of privacy. At first, he was unable to communicate his emotions to his wife. Eventually, he realized that if he did not change his rigid pattern, he would lose the relationship that he valued most. So he managed, with the support of his steady practice of Yogic ethics, to become assertive and break free of this lifelong handicap.

Both examples demonstrate the heroic capability of those who recognize that change is necessary and are brave enough to attempt it. Tolerance helps you welcome change.

Change is frightening to most people because they fear that they will lose something or suffer pain because of the change.

A STORY ABOUT TOLERANCE

The *Mahabharata* is a long epic that contains the eighteen chapters of the *Bhagavad Gita*. In this epic, there is a story about a great warrior named Bhishma that illustrates Tolerance in the heroic sense.

After the great battle that is described in the *Gita*, Bhishma lay mortally wounded, his body stuck with arrows. However, he did not want to die until the sun was in the correct position. The *Gita* talks about two paths of the sun, saying that if one dies while the sun is on its northward path (after the spring equinox), the soul has a chance to be released from the cycle of birth and death. If one dies during the southward path (after the autumn equinox), the soul is born again into the world.

Bhishma knew that he had the chance for liberation from the physical world if he could wait to die until the sun turned northward. He chose to lie on the battlefield, refusing attention to his wounds, for three months, and then gave up his body.

The physical body is naturally afraid of change. For example, if you are asked to move to a new city due to a job transfer, you may fear loss of friends or close family connections. Most fears are based on unreliable fantasies of the future or past. The practice of Tolerance helps make any place harmonious and attractive because you know the strength and steadiness that your spiritual body will supply to help you manage any changes.

Earlier I mentioned that Tolerance is often mistaken for harsh, painful austerities. People who practice this type of austerity for its own sake easily degenerate into a lifestyle of self-torture. They begin to focus on suffering to the exclusion of any other experience. There are some people who enjoy suffering. Perhaps pain is the only way for them to recognize their feel-

BE YOUR OWN BEST FRIEND

The *Bhagavad Gita* states that you are your own best friend and your own worst enemy. In my teaching, I encourage people to help themselves to grow and change in any way they can. Recognizing that there are many ways to solve problems is part of being a hero because you learn not to lock yourself into your physical body's limited point of view; instead, you enjoy the flexibility of your spiritual body's participation.

Often, students who are faced with a deep injury from the past are unable to continue happily in Yoga because all of their thoughts are spent remembering pain. Productive, creative thought is blocked, and they are unable to sustain a positive self-image. I have often advised these students to consult a professional therapist, because therapy is one way for people to regain confidence in their abilities. When this hurdle is overcome, the practice of Tolerance becomes much easier. Using every means at your disposal to help yourself is how to become your own best friend.

ings. It satisfies them in some way. This attitude, however, does not allow Tolerance to facilitate change.

The habit of suffering prevents change because people become rigid in that pattern, unable to recognize that their spiritual bodies could offer a multitude of additional options. Tolerance shows you that there are many ways to approach a difficult task and gives you the flexibility of choice. Instead of running away from your decisions in fear, you can roll up your sleeves and "go for it."

The practice of Tolerance helps you to recognize self-destructive patterns of suffering and make the choice to change. This offers you a new path to emotional freedom, because when you feel free to change and grow, your emotions (which are part of your spiritual body) are not stifled. Tolerance shows you that you can stand much more than you thought you could, including intense emotion. Thus, you no longer fear emotion.

HOW TO PRACTICE CHANGE

If you are afraid of change, try practicing change in very small, nonfrightening ways. If you wear only pastel colors, for instance, try some bright ones for a while. If you prefer chocolate ice cream, eat vanilla sometimes. Take a new route to work every so often. Keep the changes small so the experience will remain pleasant.

Small changes, practiced continually, make bigger changes easier. If, for instance, you have conditioned yourself to change your daily habits without pain, you will be better able to handle larger changes, such as a divorce, new job, or new home, with greater comfort.

After some time, the physical body will become flexible and work happily toward the freedom of expansion. When you

THE UNBURNING FIRE

A common image of purification in mythology is fire. The image is also used in discussing meditation. When there is "fuel" in the form of thoughts, the fire of the mind continues to burn. When one succeeds in thinking nothing—even for a few seconds—the fire subsides because it is not getting fuel.

Once, early in my years of practice when my first Yoga teacher, Sivananda, was alive, I had a repeating dream in which I was crawling among the timbers of the attic in a very large, empty house. The house was in flames and I was trying to find a way out. Then I saw the flames licking my legs and feet, and I realized that I felt no pain. When I asked Sivananda about this experience, he replied that there was no pain because there was no resistance.

stand secure and comfortable in the knowledge that you have the power to change, you can begin to observe the benefits of the power of Tolerance.

Freedom from the fear-of-change prison comes as a wave of confidence; eventually, you will become stable in that feeling. The feeling of confidence springs spontaneously from your spiritual body. It especially emerges when you are free to play, when you have dropped your guard. Some people are unable to play because in play, you never know what is going to happen next. Tolerance puts the fear of this type of uncertainty to rest. The new flexibility gained by Tolerance keeps you happy in unexpected circumstances.

THE POWER OF TOLERANCE

The result of practicing Tolerance was described to me by Lakshmanjoo: "Through practicing self-control and Tolerance, all impurity in your body and organs vanishes and you become filled with power."

That power is stability, knowing that you cannot be shaken. You are sure of who you are and what you want to do. It begins with the experience of an ecstacy of oneness when the physical and spiritual bodies join. Sometimes it happens in a meditative state. I first experienced this in a dream as a state of tremendous expansion. It is impossible to fully describe this dream experience, but I must say that it had a great effect on my spiritual growth. It gave me new joy in the practice of Tolerance, and I found that I had the confidence to move easily in any direction without fear.

CHAPTER 12

ETHIC #9
STUDY

Nourish Your Spiritual Body

S tudy (or *Svadyaya*, in Sanskrit) is rarely looked upon as part of ethical practice, but it can be an important source of nourishment for the spiritual body. When students ask me which sacred texts are suitable for Study, I have to say that all texts are sacred to someone like me. The practice of Yoga is not religious, and in my opinion, anything you read can be transformed into usable food for the growth of your spiritual body.

Some food is more powerful than others. I have a friend who keeps a supply of what he calls junk novels on hand for times when he feels ill or out of sorts, or for traveling. He uses this kind of Study to dull himself out and give himself a rest. It serves him by answering a specific need. All forms of Study can benefit you in some way.

HOW TO BEGIN PRACTICING STUDY

Read something every day. Choose something to read that will give enjoyment to both your physical and spiritual bodies. Pretend that you are a host expecting a very important visitor. Naturally, you wish to have the very best things at your disposal, things that your guest will enjoy. In choosing your Study materials, try to keep this attitude in mind. You do not have to read volumes; a small amount, even as little as ten to twenty minutes, is enough.

After you have finished reading for the day, take a minute to offer what you have read to your spiritual body. Start by becoming silent, and fantasize that you are making an offering of Study to your spiritual body. Ask your spiritual body if it enjoys what you have given it. This conscious connection from your physical body to your spiritual body will encourage your intuitive voice to speak.

Even ten minutes may seem an added burden to a person already working very hard and long each day, but give yourself a week's trial. Make your Study periods short and sweet. Say to yourself, "This is food that is going to comfort my inner nature. This food will satisfy my spiritual body and encourage it to show itself." Play a game with yourself. If ten minutes seems too long, promise to read just one paragraph a day. This practice will have a very quick, powerful effect, especially if you do your Study just before sleep.

I have learned to look upon Study as part of my workday. This is work that I do for myself—both of my selves. My physical body and my spiritual body both need food and attention, and Study supplies these things.

Use the ethic of Remembrance. There is a special relationship between Study and Remembrance (see chapter 13). As you study, ask yourself, "How does this relate to me? How do I feel about this?" You will get an answer from your physical body.

Now ask the same questions of your spiritual body. This will help maintain an open channel of awareness that is needed to hear the intuitive voice of the spiritual body.

Give your spiritual body enjoyable food. Many times I have seen parents place wonderful expensive food in front of children and they will not touch it. Other times I have seen a parent pick up a child and coax him to eat the plainest food and he adores it. The difference is the parent's love and attention. Your love and attention toward the spiritual body will transform what you study into the most inviting food. The way you demonstrate attention to the spiritual body is to recognize its existence and appreciate its strengths. When you develop this constant attitude, anything that you consciously offer to your spiritual body becomes enjoyable food.

The spiritual body has directed your entire life from an unseen position and is now being invited out of the darkness and onto center stage. By remembering the spiritual body's connection to you, everything that you study can become appealing to its nature. There is no need for censorship of any sort on literature, music, or any other type of expression. All expression, if offered correctly, is considered divine.

I often see people pretending to study in a thoroughly judgmental way, believing that they must either accept or reject what they read. This is your physical body trying to function alone. When you study as part of ethical practice, simply read the material, make no judgment about it, and offer it in the best, clearest condition to the spiritual body. No food that is offered with loving attention to the spiritual body is ever rejected.

When I was living in the jungle with Rama, practicing the discipline of silence, he would give me long books on classical Yoga written in Sanskrit and other languages and tell me to read them, saying, "All you have to do is look at it, and when you need to use the knowledge of the book, it will come forward." This advice has proved to be true throughout my career. Obviously, the spiritual body is a storehouse for all information.

Realize that visionary experiences do not replace Study. Sometimes I encounter people who have had marvelous visionary experiences and who conclude that they no longer need to study. Lakshmanjoo explained the problem with this point of view.

> ALICE: Sometimes people have a vision about something, so they think there is no need to study or read.
>
> LAKSHMANJOO: They are misled. There is no end. It is like . . . a blind man [who] comes to examine the body of an elephant. If he touches its leg, he says it is just like a log. He won't feel the whole of the elephant. He won't come to the real understanding of what the elephant is.
>
> ALICE: Because he has only a small picture of it.
>
> LAKSHMANJOO: Yes. That is all it is. Limited vision. As long as limited vision is existing, it is useless. It is incorrect. So you must study.

RESULTS OF PRACTICING STUDY

One of the most important functions of Study is to help you get to know yourself better by revealing your spiritual body. Study broadens your thinking and sharpens your awareness. Practice of Yoga techniques, specifically exercise, breathing, and meditation, will increase your ability to transform Study to personal experience by increasing your alertness and sensitivity, and giving you the courage to try new things.

Everything you read has meaning to the spiritual body. By offering everything to the spiritual body, you open yourself to an expansion of experience. For instance, I love to cook, so I often read cookbooks and watch cooking programs on television. When I see Julia Child using a blowtorch to light her

Cherries Jubilee, and offer what I am watching to my spiritual body, I share Julia's delight in her experience and may even consider doing something similar. If I were watching with only my physical body, I would probably dismiss the episode as a ridiculous and dangerous stunt, and I would miss the delight of a new and unusual experience.

The ability to transform what you study into something usable for both bodies is a step that is hoped for in education but is rarely taught. Most of us read and study what other people have written and use it to reinforce the outlook of our physical body instead of inviting the outlook from the spiritual body to join with us. When this relationship between the two bodies is established solidly, it will give you the power to face life with a strong, individual point of view.

THE VALUE OF SELF-UNDERSTANDING

All language is a springboard to personal experience if it is offered to both bodies. At their best, our educational systems promote this idea by stimulating students to think for themselves. All too often, however, schools, especially those for younger children, attempt to prescribe what their students should learn from their studies. Students often burn out when they try to accommodate uncounted numbers of opinions that are not their own, as if they were sophisticated memory banks.

When Study is not related to personal experience, the resulting feeling of separateness sabotages the growth of the student because it denies the participation of the spiritual body. Study helps both bodies grow and helps you discover how both bodies feel about things. Simply quoting what someone else has already said, a function of the physical body, does you little good and is, frankly, boring.

The best use of Study, then, is to help you find yourself, your reason for living, by opening you to the experience of both bodies. Lakshmanjoo translated the Sanskrit term for Study in this way.

LAKSHMANJOO: *Adyaya* means understanding; *Sva*, the self. *Svadyaya*, then, is understanding of self. Understanding of self-consciousness, through books.

ALICE: Is the self-consciousness that you're describing the same as the state of being we have discussed that is called Shiva [Universal Body]?

LAKSHMANJOO: State of being, yes.

Notice that Lakshmanjoo points out that Study is directly connected to the spiritual body, not the physical. Study is considered a food source for that body.

The problem of finding oneself is addressed in all literature. As you read, you can vicariously enjoy seeing yourself as the main characters as they struggle to accomplish this goal. Throughout this book, I have talked about the importance of fantasy techniques. Many times, the images that will illuminate your fantasies will be archetypal images, and your Study will allow you to become more familiar with these images historically and poetically. I encourage you to explore the vast array of symbolic literature that includes myths, legends, and fairy tales.

BEYOND BOOKS

All written words are observed in Yoga to be symbolic of the practice called Mantric Yoga, the repetition of a particular sound formula (given to a student by a teacher) that has a special effect on the practitioner. Mantric Yoga is considered a form of Study. Yogic cosmology states that the universe itself evolved from the primal sound "Om." This sound was given the form of a written word, and all other writing and language is supposed to have evolved from that first sound. This idea is echoed in many other creation stories around the world, such as the Bible's story of Genesis, where the "Word" is the first manifestation of God. In other words, sound took form.

A SPECIAL ASPECT
OF STUDY

There is a marvelous book called *Garland of Letters*, by Arthur Avalon, in which he discusses the Yogic philosophy of sound, writing, and language. The writing or drawing of any word is considered a *yantra*, a unique diagram that has a specific effect on the reader's brain. This special concentrative technique is also considered an aspect of Study. With the correct attention, any form of reading or writing would be considered food for the spiritual body.

ALICE: Mircea Eliade's book *Yoga, Immortality, and Freedom* says that Study consists of two things: knowledge of sciences that relate to deliverance from existence (*moksha*) and repetition of the syllable Om. Is the repetition of any or every mantram a form of Study?

LAKSHMANJOO: Only that chief mantram, Om.

ALICE: So even blind people who could not read a text could practice Study by repeating Om.

LAKSHMANJOO: Yes. I will give you a definition of Om. Om is that being, all the thirty-six elements, all these six *Kalas* [powers], six cycles, all 118 worlds. All these elements, all these worlds, and all these cycles are digested in that being of Om. And that being is not only sound. Sound is the indicator of that being. That being is bliss, *ananda*.

ALICE: By the chanting of Om, does that being eventually take form before you?

LAKSHMANJOO: It rises by and by, within oneself who is reciting this. He must know that "I am reciting this mantram Om." It is not only the word Om. It is an indicator of this being.

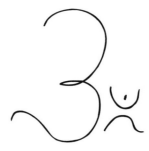

ALICE: When the syllable Om is written in Sanskrit [see illustration], what does that represent?
LAKSHMANJOO: It is a drawing of your own self. The realization of it will take place only when it is recited with great awareness and devotion.

STUDY TAKES YOU INTO SILENCE

We are used to thinking of Study as a way to understand something or to learn something—in other words, to make something our own. "Making something our own" always implies that this is being done for the use of the physical body. But when the physical and spiritual bodies work together, you will find that Study leads you to other activities, including many that you may not have considered before, such as silence. Many people do not consider silence to be an activity, but in Yoga, silence is considered an intensely energetic state.

Sometimes, you will find that when you have offered your period of Study to your spiritual body, you become filled with a deep and comforting silence. This silence clears the way for the emergence of the intuitive voice. In silence, all thinking and functioning falls away. You become aware of a marvelous feeling of expansion. The feeling is similar to what you experience in meditation when you finally succeed in stopping your inner conversation.

After this happens, your old approach to your world may seem childish, because you realize that you have been using only your physical body. Your patterns of acquiring knowledge change, and there is no limit to your mind's extension as you add the emotional, intuitive qualities of your spiritual body to the intellectual, mechanical abilities of your physical body. You are heading into the mysterious, unknown territory of your intuitive nature, inviting it to come forward with knowledge that you have never realized before, described in Shaivite philosophy as "wonder, delight, and astonishment."

CHANGING PERSPECTIVE ON WHAT YOU READ

Approaching Study with the idea of involving both bodies will change the way you perceive many things that you read. In one of my conversations with Lakshmanjoo, he discussed the Shaivite way of reading a classical text, the *Bhagavad Gita*.

> LAKSHMANJOO: Abhinavagupta has commented upon the *Bhagavad Gita* in his Shaivite book *Tantraloka*. He says, "Arjuna, trust in me. Put devotion in me. Put everything in me. I am protector of this whole world. I will protect you."
>
> ALICE: Actually, he is representing the Universal Body, isn't he? That Universal Body that supports us.
>
> LAKSHMANJOO: Yes. He has spoken in *Tantraloka* that you should not believe that Lord Krishna, in saying the word "I" in *Bhagavad Gita*, is referring to his physical body. It refers to universal God—Universal Body. It is not a person.

The word "I" in religious texts always refers to God, not a physical person. The real I, or Self, is the divine being, the Universal Body: the union of the physical and spiritual bodies. Jesus's statement "I am the Way, the Truth, and the Life" is an exact representation of this idea. The literal translation is that Jesus was talking about himself as a human person. The meaning that emerges from the spiritual body is that his use of "I" is applied to a being far beyond the physical plane—in other words, the Universal Body. Reading spiritual books in this light will give you a completely new insight into how they relate to you.

INTELLECTUAL HOARDING

Study helps you sidestep the false ego of the physical body and open the channel to the spiritual body that awaits to serve you. This would entirely do away with a demand to understand, which arises from the physical body. Such understanding would not be necessary when reliance for information is placed on the spiritual body. In fact, a demand to understand would be considered violence to the physical body because it has to strain to respond. When you feel yourself straining to understand something, the best thing to do is to become silent and fantasize the inner channel between your two bodies. This will give your physical body an immediate rest.

The principle of the ethic of Nonhoarding is clearly related to this idea. Do you study to make what you learn your own, or perhaps to gain someone else's approval? This would be considered hoarding. When you supply Study as food for your spiritual body, it would be improper to try to dictate how the spiritual body should use this food. You are simply offering it for whatever use it chooses.

When you begin to realize that a demand to understand represents intellectual hoarding by the physical body, you can immediately make a connection between your physical and spiritual bodies. When you do this, you will hear the intuitive voice of the spiritual body speak from within. In Yoga, Study is not captured and harnessed for the physical body's false ego. It is greatly respected as a power leading to freedom, an unlimited source and form that clears the channel between our two bodies. It must be given the freedom to move and change as it wishes.

REMOVING THE BLINDERS

Study broadens your capacity for experience, which promotes powerful expansion—an ability to do more and see more, as if you had removed blinders from your eyes. Hard work and Study that use only the physical body are often accompanied by headaches, fatigue, and stress. The spiritual body has no limits and does not suffer from these afflictions. It can operate tirelessly for days, years, even lifetimes. Study gives you an unlimited capacity with no effort.

Study teaches you to become an observer of yourself. You can stand slightly removed from wild, immediate, reactionary involvement with others and your surroundings, and you become able to think before you act, allowing alternative points of view into your mind. This relieves the panic-type responses that most of us experience when we think that we are going the wrong way on a one-way street.

STUDY ENCOURAGES INTUITION

Your Study provides a path that encourages full expression of the intuitive voice. The spiritual body is a storehouse for everything in this world, not only your own experiences and outlook. This remembrance reinforces the knowledge of divine sameness in all of us.

It is most interesting for me to observe my spiritual body respond with knowledge that previously seemed to be beyond my capacity. Even a small amount of training in this ethical practice will show you how to solve problems more easily. When you are presented with a problem, instead of thinking that you have to respond immediately and fix it, you can step back and wait for the spiritual body to act. And it does—very efficiently. It really surprises you because the response is delightfully different from anything you have ever seen before.

I have said that intuition is the voice of the spiritual body; you can actually hear intuition speaking. Some of you have probably experienced this spontaneously. When you Study with the idea of this extra strength behind you, intuition becomes a dependable, powerful support instead of an ethereal, unfamiliar phenomenon. I cannot remember any time in my own experience that my intuition has been incorrect. It is very comforting

LEARNING TO LISTEN
TO THE SPIRITUAL BODY

A student wrote:

The other day, I was cooking some eggs while involved in some really detailed work, and at the time, I thought to myself, "I'll bet I will forget that they are on the stove and they will overcook." Sure enough, I didn't remember the eggs until some thirty minutes later. Is there a way to stimulate my intuition to help me do multiple tasks more efficiently?

Your intuition never needs stimulation. It always stands ready to operate, but most people do not hear it when it speaks. Try to remember that it is there and ask the spiritual body to help you. It is your partner, your other half. For instance, when you put the eggs on to cook, you would say, "I don't have time to check the clock. Please tell me when the eggs are done." You will find that your intuitive voice—the voice of the spiritual body—will let you know when to check the eggs.

I use this technique all the time with many other tasks. For instance, I have not needed an alarm clock in many years. When I go to bed, I simply ask my spiritual body to wake me at a particular time, and it has never failed me. Regular practice of Study helps develop this ability to listen to your spiritual body. Try it yourself, and enjoy the delightful results.

to know that, although I may not have all the answers, something in me does.

When lecturing in South India, I often faced a double dose of hostility, because as a woman I was considered unclean, and as an American, I had no business lecturing on Yoga. My audiences often tried to confuse me by bringing up references to classical Indian texts in their questions. Although my training in those texts was not even as much as they had received at their mothers' knees, I was able to respond competently by depending upon my spiritual body to answer the question. I knew that my physical body's experience was not capable, but I was able to use my training to step aside and watch the spiritual body perform.

THE EXPANSION OF STUDY

When I feel the expansion of Study, I fantasize it as my spiritual body in full bloom, lit up with contentment, its form welcomed and encouraged to display itself freely and happily. You will notice how easy it is to do everything. The powerful personality of the spiritual body has no limit as to what it can do as the relationship between you and your spiritual body becomes solidified and comfortable.

Now it is time for you to enjoy the experience of constant change. Life loses its boring quality and becomes fresh and new. A sweet wind of freedom blows through you. The tiresome everyday existence is relieved by new opportunities. The classical texts describe the result of being established in Study as follows: "The fruit that accrues from continuously striving for self-knowledge . . . is that the Lord whom you seek will shine before you." In other words, the state of being that is the spiritual body will be visible to you in form.

CHAPTER 13

ETHIC #10
REMEMBRANCE

Recognize the Support of Your Spiritual Body

The Sanskrit term for Remembrance is *Ishwara pranidhana. Ishwara* is one name that has been given to God, which also refers to the spiritual body you're trying to invite into form by the practice of ethics. *Ishwara pranidhana*, then, means remembrance of that body with the idea that you will one day actually see the form of that body. The classical Yogic texts say that the result of practicing Remembrance is that *samadhi*—union with the divine self, or God consciousness—is quickly attained.

Remembrance is a conscious awareness that invites the practitioner to apply all the ethics in everyday life. Every action, word, thought, desire, and relationship must be examined under the bright light of ethics, and Remembrance helps you realize that you are not alone in that immense task. Remembrance is an easy way to give attention to your spiritual body so that when it appears to you, it can help you in all your endeavors.

HOW TO BEGIN PRACTICING REMEMBRANCE

Live in the moment. Remembrance is not the same as memory. Memory is our great teacher as we grow and mature in life. We can remember that putting our hand in fire is painful, so we try not to do it again. In the same way, all of our current relationships are based on our memories of what happened when we interacted with people in the past. Both past and future, then, are based on something we *already know*. This process is controlled by the physical body, and so our actions and reactions remain the same as they always have, because they are familiar.

The ethic of Remembrance, however, means something different from calling up past memories to guide our present actions. Most people believe that it is easy to remember, but you are going to be asked to remember what really hasn't happened yet. In other words, Remembrance asks you to be aware of what is happening in the present moment. Remembrance of what is happening now, in the moment, sets the scene for new and different experiences, guided by ethical behavior and supported by the spiritual body.

The practice of Remembrance gives you a wonderful experience of freedom because you are not bound by past or future behaviors. When you invite the spiritual body to guide you, you never really know what will happen next. Learning to live in the moment stops repetitive behavior, based on past memories of the physical body, that keeps you imprisoned. Whereas memory means recalling what is already known, Remembrance helps you develop the ability to face the unknown.

To pratice Remembrance, try to keep your mind centered, moving neither backward nor forward, held without inner conversation. This is similar to the practice of Contentment (see chapter 10). In that stillness, the brilliant, intuitive voice of the spiritual body may be heard. The Quakers have a similar practice, called centering, in which they quiet all actions of the body and mind and wait to hear the divine voice from within.

Begin to crack the shell of the false ego. One of the tasks of Remembrance is to learn to expand your viewpoint from the limited false ego of the physical body. A letter from a student says, "Things have gotten a bit stale with my practices." This is a common feeling for people as they begin to realize that they are basing their entire life on the limited conclusions formed by the physical body's false ego. You find yourself unable to move outside of your own circle of awareness because everything within that awareness is invented and owned by you. You get tired of hearing yourself talk.

The false ego of the physical allows no room for change. It is like riding the exercise wheel in a hamster cage, going around and around, always in the same direction, or like a crustacean that has formed a shell so tightly around itself that it becomes a boring prison. The crustacean carries its shell with it everywhere; it is the only home it knows.

For most of us, the first step in cracking the shell of the false ego is to recognize repetitive patterns in our lives. Some common examples are entering into a series of relationships with an abusive person, coping with crises by escaping through alcohol or food, and stifling feelings instead of expressing them. Take a moment to think about what patterns may be revealing themselves in your life.

If you realize that you are repeating a pattern, your first questions should be "Do I really want to do this?" and "Who is repeating this pattern?" The minute that you start this questioning, you will have started to crack your shell because you will have moved from an automatic response in your physical body (the false ego) to an observation that an unseen force is operating from the spiritual body (the true ego).

In the practice of Remembrance, you simply notice these

A TOO-COMMON FALSE EGO SHELL

The tragedy of child abuse is a prime example of how a false ego shell begins to form. When children are abused, they are unable to blame the abuser, who is often a family member, and so they blame themselves. The false ego in the child forms a shell to cope with the despair and confusion, and this shell grows as the child grows. The child becomes imprisoned in this false, egotistical outlook and the self-blame continues.

repetitive patterns without judging whether they are good or bad, and without feeling an immediate compulsion to change them. When you have the chance to examine what is happening, in light of the ethics described in this book, you will be able to see whether your patterns are destructive, or unethical in any other way, and then choose whether or not to change them.

Most people feel great relief when they realize that they no longer must bear the responsibility to fix everything that is wrong with themselves and the world. The spiritual body recognizes the fact that everything in the world is divine, not just what feels pleasant or good. This idea contrasts with religious fanaticism, in which people attempt to mold the world to fit their personal egotistical pictures. In other words, divinity lies only in what one likes. In Yogic ethics, any search for God is worthy. The idea that one search is better than another is the false ego speaking, and this type of thinking causes separation from your world and from yourself.

Welcome the unknown. We have examined how Remembrance is a practice of the present moment and how it stimulates you to break out of your limited physical body consciousness. By consciously remembering the spiritual body, you are showing attention, or devotion, to something that is currently unknown to you. You do not yet know what the spiritual body is, and you are asking it to take form so that you can get to know it.

Something similar happens in sports, music, or dance when practitioners become immersed in the experience of oneness with the movement or the sound. When this experience is realized, the way that they perform is no longer in their hands. They have prepared their physical bodies, and then, by being able to forget themselves, their spiritual bodies take over. They rest in the extraordinary position of the center. All performers are urged to use this method; it is the secret of creating an extraordinary performance.

> All great art is the work of the whole living creature, body and soul, and chiefly of the soul.
> (John Ruskin)

Imagine that you are a dancer getting ready to make an enormous leap—the perfect leap. The preparation to make that leap has become a constant desire. In fantasy, you can experience and enjoy the feeling of being airborne. In fantasy, you picture the leap, and when the fantasy takes power and form, you are able to perform it because you have opened a channel to your spiritual body.

All during your fantasy work, you are aware of your inadequacies, but success comes when you can leave them behind and launch yourself into the unknown like a pole-vaulter. You don't know what is there. You don't know if you can do it. Your fantasy allows you to begin thinking, "There is something other than what I know. I can do something more than what I can do now."

Yoga states that your personal power and ability actually extend far beyond the limits that you have placed on them through reliance on your physical body alone. By stimulating you to rest on the unknown, Remembrance becomes a bridge to truth, because the unknown is the home of your spiritual body, which can supply you with the truth in every situation.

> There is no other
> happiness here in this
> world than to be
> free of the thought
> that I am different
> from you.
> (Utpaladeva)

The spiritual body is not subject to loss, nor can it fail. So if you are feeling this way, you can use Remembrance to realize that these tendencies are simply projections from the false ego of your physical body that are building a wall of separateness between you and your own power.

LONGING FOR ONENESS WITH THE SPIRITUAL BODY

Most translations of *Ishwara pranidhana* substitute words like "worship" for Remembrance, believing that ritual, which is a large part of traditional worship, is the only type of devotion, or attention, necessary to see and interact with the spiritual body. This approach, however, implies that the spiritual body is different from you, and so perpetuates the idea that you and your spiritual body are separate. If you enjoy worship ceremonies, make them more helpful to you by constantly reminding yourself that you and the object of worship are really the same.

As you begin to feel the spiritual body's presence by using fantasy, you will realize that the spiritual body has always been there; you are simply inviting it to show itself by paying attention to it. As your fantasy of the spiritual body becomes more real to you, your inner thoughts become comments like, "How beautiful you are," or "I feel your presence," or "How wonderful it is to see you."

Many students write to me about this fantasy of the spiritual body, and I often find this plaintive statement in their letters: "I can't put this feeling into words." This statement tells me that they are filled with longing to express what is in their hearts. Many people are often filled with this sense of inexpressible longing, this feeling that something is not quite satisfied, not quite complete.

> Keep a green tree in your heart and perhaps the singing bird will come.
> (Chinese proverb)

This is a primitive feeling of longing for the spiritual body. We want to become aware of it because we know, on some level, that we are actually part of it and that it is part of us. It is difficult to articulate or even clearly identify this feeling. It is too subtle for words, but something in our physical bodies responds to this primitive longing. The practice of Remembrance helps us realize that this longing is coming from within ourselves from our spiritual nature.

Lakshmanjoo expressed it this way.

> ALICE: Why is *Ishwara pranidhana* considered to be the supreme *niyama* [observance]?
> LAKSHMANJOO: Because it is nearing end of the road. Only longing is there. Longing to hug . . .
> ALICE: The treasure?
> LAKSHMANJOO: Yes. There is one *sloka* [verse]. "When will that day come, oh Lord, when I will call you in one cry and you will be in front of me? How can I utter that kind of cry? In one cry, you will be in my arms."

The word "Lord" refers to the spiritual body, the unseen half of yourself.

BLAME GOD FOR EVERYTHING

The longing for God, or the spiritual body, gradually results in a constant Remembrance of its presence. Lakshmanjoo used to say, "Blame God for everything." He was telling me that this attitude is one way to become conscious of God in everything. By "blaming" God, or my spiritual body, for everything, I would never forget God; thus, I would always be practicing Remembrance.

> LAKSHMANJOO: There was one student who wanted to see God. His master told him, "If God does not appear to you, beat him with a stick." So there was Shiva lingam [a physical representation of the power of Shiva consciousness, usually a naturally formed phallic-shaped stone]. This student used to go and beat that lingam with his shoes. Then a flood came and this lingam was covered with water. He dived there with shoes.
>
> ALICE: To beat it some more?
>
> LAKSHMANJOO: There appeared Lord Shiva to him on that day, because he did not miss even one day. To beat him is also devotion. It is not devotion only to praise him. To beat him also is the worship. So God is never out of mind.

There is a similar thread in mythology, in stories where enemies of God are given a choice to work in an unpleasant situation acting as an adversary, and so return to God more quickly through that attitude of intense opposition, or to act as a devotee, which would mean a longer time to return to God's presence. Invariably, the adversary chooses the hostile shorter time in order to return to that beloved state of the divine as soon as possible.

The point is that such intense hostility is a type of Remembrance that can be used to bring one to ultimate realization. Whether fully agreeable or fully disagreeable, the aspirant is fully concentrated on the Remembrance of God. Lakshmanjoo and I discussed one of these stories in our conversations. (In the great epic *Ramayana*, Ravana is the demon who kidnaps Rama's wife, Sita. She is rescued, and the demon is killed by Rama, his brother Lakshmana, and the monkey god Hanuman.)

> ALICE: In mythology, there is a story about how Ravana was given a choice that he could achieve union with

SEEING GOD IN EVERYONE

Rajat Singh was one of the great kings of India. He used to wear the Kohinoor diamond on his arm, and sometimes, he hung it around his horse's neck, just for the fun of it. Any beggar who came into his court professing to have any kind of philosophical understanding was welcomed with gold dishes and jewelry and every kind of comfort, because in the Eastern way of thought, whoever comes to your door is considered divine, a representation of God that you cannot recognize but who resides in all forms of life.

So it was the custom to believe that any guest may be God taking a human form. We can never really know whom we are looking at. We may not recognize God, but the constant Remembrance that God is always there helps us to recognize the divine in all things.

Rama [another name for God] after many lifetimes of devotion or after only three lives as Rama's worst enemy. This is what you mean, isn't it? That whether you beat God or love God, it's all the same?

LAKSHMANJOO: All the same, yes, because of Remembrance.

ALICE: So, Ravana actually loved Rama?

LAKSHMANJOO: He worshipped Rama. He wanted to receive his death from Rama's sword. Otherwise, he would not have done this mischief with Sita. He would be deprived of the honor to die by Rama's hand.

ALICE: He knew Rama was going to kill him?

LAKSHMANJOO: Yes.

In this popular Indian epic, the character Ravana is depicted as practicing the greatest form of Remembrance because his constant hostility toward God was considered the same as constant devotion.

DEPENDING ON THE SPIRITUAL BODY

Practicing Remembrance gives you a support that you can always depend on. When I remember that my spiritual body is carrying all responsibility for my life, my physical body feels great relief. People find great happiness in dependence because it relieves them from carrying responsibility. But because our culture places such great value on independence, people often feel guilty about being dependent.

I have learned that there is no need to get rid of dependence. It is not inherently harmful; there is nothing wrong with it if it serves you. But I want to be dependent upon something that is real, not something that changes. I want something that lasts. For this reason, I have learned to place all dependence on my spiritual body.

The feeling of dependence that I want is similar to my experience with floating. All my life I have had the unusual ability to float in any position: vertically, horizontally, legs crossed, one arm under my head, reading books. I just don't sink. Something supports me. When I was a child, my sister used to pile stones on my stomach to see how many it would take to sink me. I can remember in India just floating along down the current on the Ganges River, and Rama running along the shore, screaming in horror, "Get out! Get out! The turtles, the turtles!" I did not know that great snapping turtles live in the northern Ganges River, feeding on corpses and ignorant swimmers.

I find great pleasure in just standing up in the water with nothing under my feet. I'm not afraid of sinking. This is the feeling of being supported totally and easily by the spiritual body. Once you feel this support, you are unafraid. You love it. What holds me up in the water? Simply the belief that I will not sink. How did I get that belief? Somehow I learned that I could be totally dependent upon an unseen support. Now I know that that support lies in my spiritual body.

REMEMBERING THE SOURCE OF EMOTION

Who makes you fall in love? Who feels love? Love makes you feel in love. It is not another person; it is love personified in the spiritual body within yourself. Love lives in the spiritual body. Love was there long before you were born and is going to be around long after you go. You can never own love—you can only experience it. When allowed, love expresses itself, and the only responsibility you have is to remember that.

Remembering that the source of such feelings is the spiritual body deepens the experience, like receiving an extra dip on an ice cream cone. This is what is meant by grace: a gift that has not been requested. The practice of Remembrance is a conscious effort to make yourself a perfect instrument for all experience. Dependence on the spiritual body is a brilliant, astonishing, nonintellectual, totally intuitive power that possesses your very being when all your walls of resistance have become porous.

> ALICE: Is devotion to God an emotional state? Is it one-pointed concentration of love, of your own desire of love for God?
>
> LAKSHMANJOO: It is intense desire. Intense desire to see him. Neglect all other things.
>
> ALICE: To someone who is aspiring . . . that is the most important thing in his life, isn't it?
>
> LAKSHMANJOO: Yes. The *only* important thing. Not most.
>
> ALICE: Everything else is just simply related to that.
>
> LAKSHMANJOO: It is just straw.
>
> ALICE: When we were talking about *Santosh* [Contentment], you said that a person must not want God consciousness. How can a person practice devotion without wanting to see God?

LAKSHMANJOO: There is urge to see him. There is not wanting. Urge to see him is in the spiritual nature. Wanting is in the physical. In wanting, there are two urgencies. Two figures which seem to be separate. A separation which does not exist.

ALICE: Is this urge coming out of one's own self?

LAKSHMANJOO: No, it is transformed. Your self is transformed in yourself.

ALICE: Into the Universal Body?

LAKSHMANJOO: Yes, because whatever exists in this universe it is not away from God consciousness, in real sense. But we don't understand that. We have neglected that side of understanding. So we think that we are kept away from God consciousness. Actually, we are not kept away from God consciousness. We have ignored God consciousness, by our own will.

When you begin to master Remembrance, you will never lose awareness of your spiritual body. The channel to your physical body will always be open. You feel a childlike wonder as the power from the spiritual body comes to you. You are not afraid in this helplessness; you feel extremely comfortable and fully supported while this change in your nature takes place. There is a great peacefulness that comes, very much like the experience that many people have described of returning to the womb, where one rests with all needs supplied, simply growing and learning, totally dependent upon the source of life in the mother. Once that peacefulness touches you, you can never forget it.

CHAPTER 14

THE PASSION
OF UNITY

Once when Rama and I were walking in his garden in the Himalayas, he pointed out a lizard that scurried away when we approached. He told me that this particular type of lizard was so poisonous that one drop of its spit could kill seven men, yet it ran away from us in fear, not remembering its power. Rama laughed and said, "You are like that, Alice!"

We are all like that lizard, in a way. Because we have forgotten our spiritual bodies, we have forgotten who we are and what we can do. It takes a special individual to look for the answer to the question "Why was I born?" One develops an overriding passion for it, a desire that supersedes everything else in life.

When I first began Yoga, I lived on the surface of my personality. My physical self, which I considered to be my entire being, was easily tired, bored, and fragile. It was not enough for me. I wanted more: more life, more knowledge, more strength, more everything. I realized that I could not do it on my own and turned to

> And when Love
> speaks, the voice of all
> the Gods makes
> heaven drowsy with
> the harmony.
> (Shakespeare, *The Two
> Gentlemen of Verona*)

my spiritual body to enlarge and brighten my world. It was a wonderful decision. My fragile physical nature turned inward to find the great power of my spiritual body waiting for me with open arms. I was continually surprised as I saw, in deep, clear flashes, that I was not at all what I seemed to be.

We became one, and from that union, I experienced a passion in life that is constantly, effortlessly reinforced and supplied from the spiritual half of my personality that never tires or dies. Passionate emotion carries us straight to the heart with no bargaining along the way. Passion is a direct route to our own emotional depth—not something reflected from some other individual, but a shining reflection of our deepest self.

The physical body connects the idea of passion with youthful sexuality, but that is only a small part of passionate experience. I can best describe passion as similar to—but far greater than—the attainment of Purity (see chapter 9): becoming one with yourself, your goals, and your life in an embrace of the physical and spiritual bodies that defines real love. A passionate person is never a watered-down personality. Most people can endure passion for only a few moments. Yogis are passionate forever.

Passionate feelings encompass my life. Everything matters to me, and because the weight of this passion is too much for me to bear in my physical body, I have to ask for extra support. That support comes from the spiritual body.

As my recognition of my spiritual body grows, I welcome the awareness that takes me out of the ordinary and into a perception of life that sings with glamour and excitement, providing a never-ending stream of knowledge and experience. This experience is available to you if you practice the ethical concepts in this book. This is the classical, well-trodden path of heroes: people who search for meaning in life. It is important to realize that whatever ethical practices you do, you are doing them for yourself alone.

> God consciousness is not achieved by means of the scriptures, nor is it achieved by the grace of your master. God consciousness is only achieved by your own subtle awareness. (Vasishtha)

The product of this ethical practice is a state known in classical Yoga as internal austerity. Most of us think of the word "austerity" as referring to some external action or discipline, but internal austerity is a state of being. It is characterized by the knowledge that you have pared yourself down so that everything has meaning to you. You have rid yourself of all unusable, unwanted, destructive parts of life; there is nothing in your life that is meaningless. In other words, you have found what you wanted and you dwell in that state, shining in simplicity, strength, and purity. You have seen yourself as you really are and you love what you see. This beautiful state of internal austerity is the source of the passion that results from the union of the physical and spiritual bodies.

The passion that lies within you is already complete. Its power does not depend on someone outside yourself. It can fully express itself in your physical body, originating from your inner divine self: your spiritual body.

Some people are afraid of passion because it sometimes seems dangerous or out of control. There is no need to be afraid. When passion is carefully guided by ethical practice, it never becomes a destroying force. It is the supplier of the beauty and depth needed to make life worth living. The passion to see and know the spiritual body brings the answer to that primitive longing for meaning, and the experience of real love blooms.

Each of us has a different capacity for passion. It is that desire to know myself, overriding everything else, that has brought me to Yoga. The heart knows what it wants, and it is up to you to clear the path for its fulfillment. The ethical principles of Yoga allow that path to be cleared safely. It is not always easy, but those of you with depth of passion will do it anyway, because, in the end, you find that you cannot do anything else.

THE ROSE-COLORED GLASSES

Are you familiar with the famous story of the rose-colored glasses? A man walks into an old, dusty antique shop and sees a pair of rose-colored glasses. He puts them on and realizes that he suddenly knows what everybody is thinking.

He buys the glasses and goes out into the world, using them to become tremendously successful, wealthy, and powerful. In spite of this, however, happiness eludes him. Life is too simple. There is no fun of failure, winning or losing. He knows that he cannot fail. And so he puts the glasses in the top drawer of his dresser, thinking that he does not need them anymore because he has everything the world can give him.

A long time later, however, some crisis happens. He realizes that he needs the glasses again and runs upstairs to rummage through his dresser. He finds the glasses, frantically puts them on, and happens to glance in the mirror at his own reflection. Suddenly, he sees himself—and he collapses and dies in shock. The glasses allow him to see himself as he really is, and he cannot stand it.

As we become more familiar with ourselves, the experience can sometimes be as frightening as it is compelling, because we are not used to examining ourselves so closely. We are not used to seeing our struggles and powers in such direct light. The practice of ethics and the remembrance of the spiritual body provide a cushion for those unknown qualities as they gradually become revealed to us. A student wrote to me about this experience.

I recently noticed a wonderful break in a rigid pattern of thinking that has been with me my entire life. When working with other people, I used to be unable to consider any option besides the one that seemed most "logical" to me. People often got very frustrated with me because whenever they offered a suggestion, my automatic response was "no."

As I started to become more aware of what I was doing, because of my practice of Yogic ethics, I began to realize that this rigid pattern was violating all sorts of ethics: Nonviolence, Nonhoarding, and Contentment are just a few that come to mind. For a while, I became deeply troubled—almost depressed—because this rigidity seemed so deeply ingrained that I despaired of ever changing it, even though I was trying so hard to be ethical.

One day, I was thinking about something you said, and I finally realized that in taking on the responsibility for changing this pattern myself, I was using only my physical body. I decided to try your fantasy exercise of asking my spiritual body for help with this problem.

The very first time I tried it, I had written a press release and was going over it with my boss. I started to feel the familiar stubbornness when my boss suggested some changes, but I remembered the technique and asked my spiritual body to help out. I found myself really listening for once, instead of immediately objecting. And then a thought came to me—I guess my intuition—suggesting a way to word the paragraph in question so that both of our concerns were addressed. I felt almost lightheaded with happiness, as if a door had opened within me and a bright light was shining through.

This is why the practice of ethics is so important: It provides a cushion of protection from, and guidance in, the force of change.

WHEN A GURU APPEARS

A passionate desire for meaning in life, guided by careful, steady training in ethical behavior, produces a new individual, born again, a mystic. I use the term mystic in the traditional sense, of one who has knowledge of spiritual truth and a feeling of unity with the divine. This ecstatic existence is so complicated that it is impossible to intellectually understand it, but it can be experienced.

When an individual has a passionate desire to experience this ecstasy, usually a teacher or a guru appears in his or her life. They move on together toward the ultimate goal of union with the inner divine self. The saying is often quoted: "When the student is ready, the guru appears." The next sentence, rarely acknowledged, is "One gets the guru one deserves."

Until a guru appears, the best thing to do is to simply follow the ethical principles outlined in this book. By doing this, it will be easy to place more reliance on your inner power, and you can gradually begin to experience the confidence and happiness of knowing that your life is fully supported.

In Indian art, there are many images of Shiva, which we have discussed as representing a state of consciousness. He is often shown in the form of an ascetic, seated in meditation, with the Ganges River pouring down upon his head. Shiva deflects the power of the river's force by diverting the rush of water through his long, matted locks so that the earth is not injured by the impact of the flood. In this image, the river depicts the force of the unknown self as the channel between the physical body and the spiritual body is opened, and Shiva's head represents the protective quality of the practice of ethics.

THE EXCITEMENT
OF UNCERTAINTY

Once you realize that another source of life lies within you, the enjoyment of watching your spiritual body's form emerge becomes a continual occupation. I have tried to get to know that other half of myself intimately. It always knew me; it was part of me, but I had not recognized it. Now I find that I am very rarely bored, and I have great strength because I am no longer only "half there." The frustration of feeling constantly limited by what I know is gone, as I have learned to depend more and more upon what I do not know. My unconscious has come forward to show its tremendous capacity, and I incorporate its abilities into my everyday life.

I realize that my spiritual body is the heart of all my emotions and is the direct, clear voice in my intuition. Before I practiced Yoga, I would many times ignore my intuition, hearing it speak but trying not to pay too much attention to it. Now I know that I can depend on it completely, and I wait to hear its voice before making any decisions. It is fun to do, playing and fantasizing with all the possibilities. When any decision is to be made, no matter how small, I find that I can quickly decide what "I" want to do, but I wait to see what "it"—my spiritual body—wants to do.

In the beginning, it slowed me down a bit, but I have found this attitude very protective for me in that I have learned to make very few impulsive decisions. I do not feel impatient at the wait that is needed for answers from both bodies. In fact, I feel much more secure and confident that my whole being is involved in actions guarded by tolerance, restraint, and the extra input of information that comes from a fully functioning intuition and ethical behavior.

There is no fear in meeting with the unknown for me. I have no fear of losing or the humiliation of failure. Life is always more interesting when you do not know what will happen next. Rama was like that. He would sit in class with students and say, "Ask me something! Ask me anything!" Not at all afraid that he would give the wrong answer, he knew that the words he spoke would surprise him because they came from the intuitive voice of the spiritual body, the source of the unknown. He was ready for anything that it could tell him because he had prepared the way, designing a strong, guarded path that protected him from all harm.

Lakshmanjoo once said, "Once you're on a path, you can't get off it." It becomes a burr under your saddle. I cannot say that you're going to like it or hate it or enjoy it or love it; it simply exists. But I can tell you that it has been the reason for my existence all my life. Every day, I find myself respectfully asking my spiritual body to show itself in all its power, saying, "I must know! I must see you!" And I have never regretted it for a moment.

RESOURCES FROM THE
AMERICAN YOGA
ASSOCIATION

For further information on Yoga, including a complete catalog of the books and tapes described below, or for information about classes in Sarasota, Florida, please send a self-addressed, stamped envelope to the American Yoga Association (AYA), 513 South Orange Avenue, Sarasota, FL 34236.

For information on classes in the Cleveland area, write to the American Yoga Association, P.O. Box 18105, Cleveland Heights, OH 44118.

BOOKS

20-Minute Yoga Workouts: The Perfect Program for the Busy Person. Brief routines that anyone can fit into the busiest schedule. Includes chapters on women's issues, toning and shaping, the "twenty-minute challenge," and away-from-home workouts.

The American Yoga Association Beginner's Manual. Complete instructions for more than ninety Yoga exercises and breathing techniques; also includes three ten-week curriculum outlines and chapters on nutrition, philosophy, stress management, sports, and pregnancy.

The American Yoga Association's New Yoga Challenge. The chapters in this book—Attention, Energy, Strength, Flexibility, Steadiness, and Focus—introduce different approaches for achieving oneness of body and mind through challenging physical workouts and creative philosophical concepts. The concluding chapter, The Powerful Individual, shows you how to design your own routine according to your needs, goals, and tendencies.

The American Yoga Association Wellness Book. A basic routine to maintain health and well-being, this book also includes chapters on how Yoga can specifically help with fifteen common health conditions, among them arthritis, heart disease, back pain, premenstrual syndrome, menopause, weight management, insomnia, and headaches.

Conversations with Swami Lakshmanjoo, Volume I: Aspects of Kashmir Shaivism. Edited transcripts of Alice Christensen's interviews with Swami Lakshmanjoo, talking about his childhood and early years in Yoga, plus some basic concepts in the philosophy of Kashmir Shaivism.

Conversations with Swami Lakshmanjoo, Volume II: The Yamas and Niyamas of Patanjali. Edited transcripts of Alice Christensen's dialogues with Swami Lakshmanjoo about these essential ethical guidelines in Yoga.

Easy Does It Yoga. For seniors or those with physical limitations due to illness, injury, substance abuse recovery, obesity, or chronic inactivity, this book includes instruction in breathing techniques, meditation, and specially adapted Yoga exercises that can be done in a chair or in bed.

Easy Does It Yoga Trainer's Guide. A complete manual for how to begin teaching the Easy Does It Yoga program to seniors or others with physical limitations. Excellent for health professionals, activities directors, physical therapists, home health aides, and others who work with the elderly or in rehabilitative services.

The Joy of Celibacy. This book examines how the unconscious is influenced by the sexual sell of modern advertising and suggests a five-minute celibacy break to help build awareness and self-knowledge. (soon to be published)

The Light of Yoga. A chronicle of the unusual circumstances that catapulted Alice Christensen into Yoga practice in the early 1950s, including the teachers and experiences that shaped her first years of study.

Meditation. A collection of excerpts from Alice Christensen's lectures and classes on the subject of meditation, including a section of questions and answers from students.

Reflections of Love. A collection of excerpts from Alice Christensen's lectures and classes on the subject of love.

AUDIOTAPES

Complete Relaxation and Meditation with Alice Christensen. A two-tape audiocassette program that features three guided meditation sessions of varying lengths, including instruction in a seated posture, plus a discussion of meditation experiences.

The "I Love You" Meditation Technique. This technique begins with the experience of a more conscious connection with the breath through love. It then extends this feeling throughout the body and mind in relaxation and meditation. This tape teaches you the beauty of loving yourself and it removes unseen fear.

VIDEOTAPES

Basic Yoga. A complete introduction to Yoga that includes exercise, breathing, and relaxation and meditation techniques. Provides detailed instruction in all the techniques, including variations for more or less flexibility, plus a special limbering routine and back-strengthening exercises. Features a thirty-minute practice session in a Yoga class setting for a convenient daily routine.

Conversations with Swami Lakshmanjoo. A set of three videotapes in which Alice Christensen introduces Swami Lakshmanjoo and talks with him about his background, the philosophy of Kashmir Shaivism, and other topics in Yoga. (Some material corresponds to Volume I of the book *Aspects of Kashmir Shaivism.*)

The Hero in Yoga: A Videotape Study Program. A series of twenty-four videotaped lectures by Alice Christensen on Joseph Campbell's landmark text *The Hero with a Thousand Faces,* showing how the adventure of the hero, represented in mythologies all over the globe, parallels the Yoga student's search for self-actualization.

The Yamas and Niyamas: A Videotape Study Program. A series of twenty-five videotapes of Alice Christensen's comprehensive lectures on the ethical guidelines that form the cornerstone of Yoga philosophy and practice.

CREDITS

The excerpts from the Upanishads on pages 6 and 22 are from *The Upanishads: Breath of the Eternal*, translated by Swami Prabhavananda and Frederick Manchester (Vedanta Press, 1957).

The excerpt from Utpaladeva's poem on page 174 is from *Shaiva Devotional Songs of Kashmir*, translated by Constantina Rhodes Bailey (SUNY Press, 1987).

The excerpts from the *Rig Veda* on page 3 are from *Vision of the Vedic Poets*, translated by Jan Gonda (Mouton de Gruyer, 1960).

The quotation from Abhinavagupta on page 7 is from *The Triadic Heart of Shiva*, translated by Paul Muller-Ortega (SUNY Press, 1989).

All quotations from the *Bhagavad Gita* are from the Gita Press edition, translated by Jayadayal Goyandka, 1975.

ABOUT THE AMERICAN
YOGA ASSOCIATION

The American Yoga Association teaches a comprehensive and balanced program of Yoga exercise, breathing, and meditation. Rather than focusing primarily on physical conditioning, our core curriculum acknowledges the deeper possibilities of Yoga and encourages the inner-directed awareness that eventually leads to greater self-knowledge. This reliance on individual experience and feeling is a central theme in the science of Yoga, and it underlies the philosophical system of Kashmir Shaivism, which supports our line of teaching.

ABOUT THE AUTHOR

Alice Christensen stands out as a Yoga teacher with the rare ability to make the often-complex ideas and techniques of Yoga accessible to our Western outlook and lifestyle. She established the American Yoga Association in 1968, which was then the first and only nonprofit organization in the United States dedicated to education in Yoga.

Alice has consistently presented Yoga in a clear, classical manner for over forty years. She presents Yoga without dogma or prescription, as a potent avenue for individual inquiry, in formats that can be used to enhance any lifestyle. Whether the goal is to maintain health or to explore the nature of the self, her programs can be used to achieve a wide range of goals.

INDEX